Handbook of
Pediatric Physical
Diagnosis

D0959431

Handbook of Pediatric Physical Diagnosis

Lewis A. Barness, M.D.
Professor of Pediatrics
College of Medicine
University of South Florida
Tampa, Florida

**FOREWORD BY
David S. Cooper, M.D.**
Resident Physician
Department of Pediatrics
College of Medicine
University of South Florida
Tampa, Florida

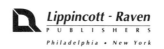

Lippincott - Raven
PUBLISHERS
Philadelphia • New York

Acquisitions Editor: Paula Callaghan
Developmental Editor: Lesa Ramsey
Manufacturing Manager: Dennis Teston
Production Manager: Robert Pancotti
Production Editor: Jeff Somers
Indexer: Lisa Mulleneaux
Compositor: Circle Graphics
Printer: R. R. Donnelley

Printed in the United States of America

9 8 7 6 5 4 3 2 1

Library of Congress Cataloging-in-Publication Data

Handbook of pediatric physical diagnosis / editor, Lewis A. Barness;
    foreword by David S. Cooper.
        p.   cm.
    Includes bibliographical references and index.
    ISBN 0-7817-1682-9 (alk. paper)
    1. Children—Medical examinations.   2. Children—Diseases—
Diagnosis.   3. Physical diagnosis.   I. Barness, Lewis A.
    [DNLM: 1. Physical Examination—in infancy & childhood—handbooks.
WS 39 H2362 1998]
RJ50.H365   1998
618.92′0075—dc21
DNLM/DLC
for Library of Congress

Care has been taken to confirm the accuracy of the information presented
and to describe generally accepted practices. However, the author and
publisher are not responsible for errors or omissions or for any consequences
from application of the information in this book and make no warranty,
express or implied, with respect to the contents of the publication.
    The author and publisher have exerted every effort to ensure that drug
selection and dosage set forth in this text are in accordance with current
recommendations and practice at the time of publication. However, in view of
ongoing research, changes in government regulations, and the constant flow
of information relating to drug therapy and drug reactions, the reader is
urged to check the package insert for each drug for any change in indications
and dosage and for added warnings and precautions. This is particularly
important when the recommended agent is a new or infrequently employed
drug.
    Some drugs and medical devices presented in this publication have Food
and Drug Administration (FDA) clearance for limited use in restricted
research settings. It is the responsibility of the health care provider to
ascertain the FDA status of each drug or device planned for use in their
clinical practice.

Contents

Foreword

See what everyone else has seen,
but think what no one else has thought—Anonymous

Dramatic changes have occurred in the care of children since Dr. Barness first published his *Manual of Pediatric Physical Diagnosis* in 1957. Despite the advent of powerful technologies, the cornerstone of patient care still remains the history and physical examination. In this era of lab tests, though, it seems the importance of the physical exam has been "forgotten."

In a medical education system that is dominated by "adult" medicine, the special approach to unique physical examination techniques in infants and children is often lost. This is compounded by the fact that no book dedicated entirely to the examination of the pediatric patient is currently available.

Manual of Pediatric Physical Diagnosis has, since its inception, served to educate its audience about the examination of the pediatric patient in an objective, analytical, and humanistic manner. It makes us privy to the lifetime experiences of Dr. Barness via an organ system–oriented approach to the examination of the patient. With this new version, new charts and diagrams have been added as well as tables containing pertinent differential diagnoses of both common and rare conditions.

It has been both a pleasure and an honor to participate in the review and editing of this outstanding manual. Anyone involved in the care of infants and children will only benefit from the wisdom and experience this book can teach.

David S. Cooper
Resident Physician
University of South Florida

Preface

In pediatric practice, there is no substitute for the physical examination. A thorough physical, along with a complete history, is still the best basis for most diagnosis. When dealing with infants, children, and adolescents, "laying on of the hands" is crucial if one is to provide effective and productive care. As the focus in the classroom, examination room, and medical literature shifts to computers, technical devices, and sophisticated laboratory tests, the importance and necessity of the comprehensive physical diagnosis and detailed history can sometimes be overlooked. This combination of incomplete physical exam and history and increased use of modern devices (along with the pressures of cost containment and shortened contact time) has led to complaints of coldness on the part of the physician. For the physician treating the pediatric patient, it is especially important to avoid this trend. The practice of "laying on of the hands" is a fundamental component of diagnosis. Patients and parents want a physician who can use not only the latest technological diagnostic tools but also the "old-fashioned" methods for arriving at a diagnosis. For the practicing pediatrician, physical examinations and "laying on of the hands" can lead to greater personal rewards and gratification.

This new edition of the *Handbook of Pediatric Physical Diagnosis* provides the student and practitioner with an extensive review of the special methods used in pediatric physical diagnosis. The reader will find various sections that discuss the characteristics and specifics of the physical examination, including the approach to the patient, the examination of the body, the neurologic examination, and the examination of the newborn. In addition, the requests and suggestions of readers and residents have been incorporated in this edition, resulting in revisions and updates to most of the text and more of the information (particularly of diagnoses) appearing in table and list form.

For this edition, as with the volumes in the past, I am grateful to many people for their comments and criticisms, particularly my wife, Enid. David Cooper, a resident who has read the entire volume, also made numerous useful suggestions and has written a foreword to this edition. Dr. John Silverio, a colleague, and John Bohn, a former resident, again gave many helpful suggestions. I also want to thank my grandchildren, who continue to provide new challenges in diagnosis. In addition, Lesa Ramsey of Lippincott–Raven Publishers has been most helpful in the development of this text. I am especially grateful to Paula Callaghan of Lippincott–Raven Publishers for her editorial suggestions and for returning the manual to pocket size. Finally, thanks to my secretary, Rebecca Scott, who has tolerated numerous editions and revisions.

I hope this volume will help improve the care of children.

Introduction

A complete physical examination in a child emphasizes many characteristics that differ from those in adults. It is important to recognize these differences and also the many variations among normal children.

This is a manual of the special methods used in pediatric physical diagnosis. It is assumed that the person using it has the basic knowledge of physical examination of adults, for which many textbooks have been written. Therefore no extensive details are listed of the definition of a sign or of methods of eliciting a sign unless special methods are used in children. Although the material in this manual includes only the actual physical examination, diagnoses cannot be made by physical examination alone. Before the examination is started, it is important that a careful and detailed history must be taken of the patient and family and that this be made part of the patient's record. As the art of careful observation is learned, diagnosis by physical examination becomes easier. In younger children from whom no history can be directly obtained, or in the child whose parents lack the ability of accurate observation, this is indeed necessary.

Examples of disease states are given throughout this manual. At no time are these states to be considered the complete differential diagnosis of the sign given. The examples are given only to present a better understanding of the sign under discussion. The beginner may use this manual to learn to elicit a particular sign; the disease states indicated will later have meaning.

If further examples of a sign are desired, standard references are suggested. The references used freely in the development of this manual include the easily available standard pediatric texts.

Many suggestions have been made for improvement of this manual by students, house officers, and physicians. Especially important are the suggestions offered by Dr. David Cooper, who critiqued the entire manuscript but who has made the suggestion that more lists be included of diseases, which in previous editions were presented in cursive style. We hope that this will improve readability, but should not be construed as a complete list of differential diagnoses.

There is no "routine" physical examination of a child. Each examination is individualized. Not only are there many physical differences that an examiner accustomed to adults might consider abnormal in a child but also the variations among a group of children make the examiner more alert to the broad spectrum included in the term "normal." The physician adept at physical diagnosis in children is one who is aware of these variants.

Most of the observed variations can best be explained by the difference in growth rates of the organ systems as they occur from infancy to maturity. For example, the lymphoid tissue is relatively well developed in infancy, becomes maximally developed during childhood, and regresses to small adult proportions at puberty. The nervous system, on the other hand, is largely developed at birth and reaches almost complete adult size by age 5 years. The genital system, however, is infantile until puberty. These and other variations will be noted throughout the discussion of the physical examination.

A mother frequently asks: "Is my child normal?" With only a single observation of a child one is rarely able to tell whether or not the child is entirely normal, though one may frequently be able to tell that the child is abnormal. Normality in pediatrics, as in statistics, is often confused with the average, and statisticians conclude that considerable variation from the average exists in any normal static population. Normality in children includes the many differences existing at about the average of the age of the child being studied, with adequate consideration of the child's background and environment. Determining normality in an ever-changing individual is even more difficult. In conducting a physical examination, one seeks normal, variations from normal, and abnormal states. One also determines the general mental and physical state, congenital and acquired anomalies, and pathologic or disease states.

The record of a complete physical examination in children has special importance not found in that of adults. This record of examination represents a report of one specific time in a child's life when that child is continually and rapidly changing. Therefore it will be used as a basis for determining whether that child is growing and developing normally, according to a group of standards learned from books, mothers, and patients. More important than a single observation of the child is the use made of this record in following the *rate* of change of the child at each subsequent examination. The rate of growth, rate of development, and, indeed, rate of progression of difficulties or anomalies far surpass for evaluation purposes the single examination. The single examination is valuable, of course, not only for determining acute illnesses but also for determining for the physician, parent, and child the gross evaluation of the potentialities and liabilities of the child. Therefore, even small and apparently insignificant variants should be noted for each child so that their importance may be adequately assessed in later examination.

For example, if a child with nausea and vomiting was adequately examined 2 weeks before the illness and the liver was not palpable at the time but is now palpable 2 cm below the right costal margin, one should direct attention to the liver as a possible cause of the illness. In contrast, if the child's liver was palpable 2 weeks before the acute illness, the now palpable liver requires less attention. This type of notation is especially important for so-called innocent murmurs of childhood, which are notorious for their frequent change, the significance of which may take many months and many examinations to determine.

The physical examination of a child should also constitute a record that can be easily interpreted by other physicians. Appendix A contains a form for recording a physical examination. Although the method of recording the physical examination is a logical order, the examination itself is not necessarily performed in that order.

Approach to the Patient

More is missed by not looking than by not knowing.

All doctors have series of tricks of examination that they have developed with experience. You may gain the cooperation of older children by making flattering remarks about their clothing or by holding conversations on their level and discussing mutual interests. You may reassure and distract preschool children with interesting objects. Frequently, a 2- to 4-year-old child will remain quiet and apparently interested if you start a pointless story, particularly about imaginary animals, and ask the child equally pointless questions about these animals. With infants, you must sometimes resort to physical measures such as sugar-feeding to keep them quiet. Even a 2-year-old child may respond to flattery; a 3- to 6-year-old may enjoy being told he looks like a 7- to 10-year-old and, although bribery of any kind is normally deplorable, a judiciously offered lollipop may create an everlasting attachment between patient and physician.

Usually, the examination of infants or preteens is performed while the parent is present. If the child is frightened or clings to the parent, sending the parent out of the room usually serves only to frighten the child more. Failure of a child aged 4 years or more to cooperate reasonably well is evidence of something abnormal in your approach or in the child's past experience or personality. On rare occasions, you may ask the parent to leave the room, but you should do this before performing the examining. Ask adolescents if they desire a parent to be present. If not, a chaperone of the appropriate sex should be present. Before beginning the examination, always wash your hands with warm water. This serves to cleanse and warm the hands so that the patient will not be uncomfortable. The parents also become aware of your consideration and appreciate routine hand washing. If the mother stands at the examining table, she should be at the child's feet. Organize your approach so that each part of the body is examined only once.

In general, begin the physical examination using no instruments and gradually introduce the various necessary examining equipment. You can frequently make a tentative diagnosis by observing the young child either while the child is in the mother's arms or is walking or standing in the room. This diagnosis can be confirmed after a thorough examination is made. Usually, infants are examined in a crib or on a table. The examining table or bed should be large enough that children will have no fear of falling and high enough that the physician can examine them in comfort.

Physical examinations are performed on children by taking full advantage of opportunities as they present themselves. Physicians concerned with the physical and mental habits of children realize that they must use all their wiles to establish rapport. The order of an adequate examination is therefore determined more by the child than by the physician.

The examination is usually performed with patients in the position most suitable to them. For the most part, infants, severely ill children, or children who understand well may be conveniently examined in the supine position. However, a 6-month-old child may have just learned to sit up and may be anxious to demonstrate this ability. Therefore, the examination should be performed chiefly with the patient in the sitting position. Similarly, some children may prefer being examined while standing or in unusual positions; the physician should respect such preferences if they do not interfere with a complete examination. It is especially important that children with respiratory distress be examined in the position of most comfort that provides the best airway: usually a sitting or sometimes a prone position.

An obstreperous or frightened patient, however, may reject all attempts at examination. Frequently, even this kind of patient can be examined completely while being held in the mother's arms. This is the position of preference especially for many children aged 1 to 3 years. Other children may have the ears or mouth examined while being held by the mother. If the patient clings to the mother, the back and extremities may be examined in this position and the remainder of the examination can be performed later with the patient supine. Examining the abdomen of a child held in the mother's lap is usually unsatisfactory. If the mother is helping restrain the patient, she should be told to hold the patient's hands rather than arms. If she holds the arms, the patient's hands are free to interfere with you.

Restraining the patient to examine such parts as the ears or mouth may occasionally be necessary. Place the infant's arms under the back so that the infant's weight rests on the palms. You or the mother can restrain the infant's head, and the examination can proceed.

Aware that the sight of many instruments may frighten the child, most pediatricians start the physical examination with observation of the hands and feet and then the chest or abdomen. They then auscultate, percuss, and palpate these areas and proceed with the remainder of the examination. The genitalia, femoral areas, and anus can be examined next in boys and younger girls, but these areas are examined last in older girls. Next, it is usually convenient to examine the head, eyes, face, and neck and then the ears, nose, and throat. In older girls, the labia and introitus are then examined. Determining blood pressure and other measurements and testing mass reflexes concludes the examination in younger children. In older children and teens, one first determines blood pressure and other measurements, and then proceeds with the examination from the head downward systematically, as in adults. While you perform the examination, it often helps if you allow the patient to play with the instruments you are going to use or have just finished using. When cooperation is desired for the difficult procedures, *tell* patients firmly what they are to do rather than *ask* them to do something.

Before you contemplate performing a frightening or painful procedure, tell patients what is to be done and what is expected of them. Reserve procedures such as examination of the head (during which instruments are inserted into the ears and mouth) and the rectum for the end of the examination in young children. Rectal examination is done whenever the patient has any symptom referable to the gastrointestinal tract. If children are old enough to understand, tell them that these procedures are "uncomfortable but not painful."

Any discomfort caused a patient should last as short a time as possible. If you feel that at any time in the examination you must hurt the patient, do not tell the patient otherwise during the visit. If the child is acutely ill or hyperirritable, take little time for the amenities and proceed rapidly with the examination.

Occasionally, especially in acutely ill patients, you may have suspicions regarding a particular diagnosis and may wish to confirm or eliminate this diagnosis before proceeding with the examination. For example, if meningitis is suspected in an infant, you may palpate the fontanel first, or if acute abdomen or congenital heart disease is suspected, you may examine the abdomen or heart first. You must be cautious in following such a procedure in patients who are not as acutely ill. Too frequently, a relatively unimportant secondary diagnosis may be found, and you may forget to complete the examination that would reveal the primary diagnosis.

You must also be cautious in following this procedure in children with obvious skin blemishes or other gross deformities or in those with suspected psychiatric difficulties or mental deficiency. In such children, examining first those areas in which difficulty is *not* expected avoids drawing the attention of the child or parent to the obvious difficulty.

Ordinarily, an experienced physician should take no longer than 5–10 minutes to perform a complete physical examination. Speed is necessary to avoid exhausting the patient. At each visit, regardless of the patient's chief complaint or reason for the visit, you should perform a complete systematic examination and record any abnormalities. Few doctors miss diagnoses because of ignorance; errors are caused by careless omission of simple procedures.

During each examination, the child should be completely undressed so that the entire body may be examined. If the room is cool or if the patient is modest or frightened, first part of the child's clothing may be removed and replaced and then another. The degree of modesty varies greatly among children, and modesty should be respected in a child regardless of age.

Above all, successful doctors caring for children must obtain genuine pleasure from examining and dealing with them. They should be friendly and unharried and must proceed with the examination with interest, patience, dexterity, and confidence. Children respond well to physicians who demonstrate confidence, and parents are more likely to accept diagnoses and treatment from physicians who are thorough.

Measurements, Vital Signs

The usual measurements taken during a physical examination include temperature, pulse rate, respiratory rate, height, weight, and blood pressure. For children aged less than 2 years, the circumference of the head, chest, and abdomen should also be measured. Other measurements, such as pelvic width, crown–rump distance, waist and hip circumference, and sitting and standing height, are ordinarily not determined in the physical examination unless the physician suspects abnormalities.

TEMPERATURE

The patient's temperature is best taken either immediately before the physical examination is started or after it is completed. Temperatures are probably of more value to parents than to physicians. If a patient is ill, 1 degree more or less of fever does not mean one degree more or less of disease. However, parents like to know how many degrees of fever their child has and are reassured if the child's temperature is normal.

Obtain a satisfactory routine temperature in a child aged less than 6 years by placing the thermometer in the axilla or groin, placing the arm or the leg along the patient's body, and holding the arm or leg against the thermometer for 3 minutes. In general, axillary or groin temperatures are about 2 degrees lower than rectal temperatures and 1 degree lower than oral temperatures.

If you wish to determine an infant's temperature rectally, grease the thermometer well and insert it past the mercury bulb. Place the infant face down across the mother's lap with the legs dangling along the mother's leg. The mother should hold the infant's buttocks firmly with one hand and the arm of that hand should lie firmly across the infant's back. The thermometer is inserted about 2 cm and should be held by the parent or you as long as it is in place. Do not attempt to take a rectal temperature in children who have rectal diseases or vulvovaginitis; note that rectal temperatures are more frequently elevated after exercise than are oral temperatures. Never take rectal temperatures in a child lying supine because the thermometer will be inserted at the wrong angle, increasing the chances of breaking the thermometer or perforating the rectum.

Newborns may have an axillary temperature of 33°–36°C. Only after 1 week is the temperature stabilized at 36°C axillary.

Do not take oral temperatures until children understand what is expected of them, which usually occurs after age 6 years. The newer electronic thermometers are rapid and accurate and can be used in any orifice regardless of a child's age.

Fever is a manifestation of increased metabolism and may be caused by a variety of disorders. In children, a body temperature of 40°–40.5°C corresponds approximately to a temperature of 38.5°–39°C in adults. Children normally may have elevated temperatures after eating or vigorous play, in the afternoon, or when excited. Children aged 6 or even 8 years of age frequently have temperature elevations to 40°C with minor or major bacterial, viral, and protozoan infections, with dehydration, or with heat stroke. Upper respiratory infections or kidney infections in infants or sinusitis, otitis, or prodromal stages of infectious diseases in older children are particular infections that may be difficult to determine on examination but that frequently cause fever.

Fever may also be evident in children with brain injury, particularly cerebral hemorrhage or brain tumor, in those with maldevelopment of the brain, and in those who are unable to sweat because of poisoning (especially atropine) or ectodermal dysplasia. Transfusion reactions, intravascular hemolysis or inflammation, and sickle cell crisis may be accompanied by fever. Large daily temperature variations are sometimes noted with septicemia, liver or kidney disease, tumors, rheumatoid arthritis, Hodgkin's disease, and leukemia. Persistent low-grade temperature elevations to 39°C are common in rheumatic fever and other collagen-vascular disorders but may also occur in other conditions.

Temperature elevations above 40°C (axillary), especially if the rate of elevation is rapid, are sometimes accompanied by seizures in young children with no other evidence of convulsive disorders. A temperature elevation of this degree in a child who looks well, is playing, and has no obvious disease may indicate the presence of roseola infantum.

Hypothermia is usually due to chilling but also occurs in shock states. Especially in infants, however, a normal or low body temperature is common despite overwhelming infections.

PULSE

Obtain a pulse rate in young infants, by either palpation or auscultation over the heart and in older children by palpation at the wrist or at other sites (see Chapter 5). The significance of the pulse rate, rhythm, and quality is discussed in the section on examination of the heart.

RESPIRATORY RATE

Obtain the respiratory rate by watching, palpating, or auscultating the chest. In young children, accurate respiratory rates can be obtained only during sleep. The significance of the respiratory rate is discussed in the section on examination of the lungs. Children with a rapid respiratory rate usually have respiratory distress or severe infection, and children with a slow respiratory rate usually are free of respiratory difficulty.

HEIGHT

The height or length of the child, together with the weight, is not only a good measure of the overall growth of the child but also provides a record of the rate of growth for easy comparison with children of similar stature and age as recorded in standard charts. One prime characteristic that distinguishes a child from an adult is increasing growth; if you note failure of growth, suspect some difficulty in the development of the child (see Appendix C).

Measure the infant supine. Hold the zero end of the tape at the infant's heel and read the marking at the infant's head to the nearest centimeter. Older children can be measured standing on the scale. At this time, recording the approximate height of parents and grandparents is also of value. The most common cause of unusual growth apparently is genetic influence. Although height is not strictly inherited, tall parents tend to have taller children than short parents.

If broad allowances are made for normal variations and the child still appears abnormal in height, consider the variations in time of growth. Some children grow rapidly at one age and more slowly at another, and these growth spurts may not correspond to the average. If growth still appears abnormal, seek other explanations.

Abnormal *shortness*, as determined by charts with standard deviations, may be caused by any chronic disease affecting absorption or utilization of nutrients.

Malnutrition

Deprivation	Inflammatory bowel disease
Food fads	Gastrointestinal malformation
Cystic fibrosis	Vitamin deficiencies
Food allergy	Mineral deficiencies
Celiac disease	Developmental delay
Hemolytic anemias	

Dwarfism may also be due to the chondrodystrophies or other diseases involving the spine; in some cases, no cause may be found.

Growth Retardation

Genetic	Russell-Silver syndrome
Chromosomal	de Lange syndrome
Familial	Prader-Willi syndrome
Chondrodystrophies	Skeletal dysplasias
Growth hormone deficiency	Hypercorticism
Thyroid deficiency	Precocious puberty
Diabetes	Hypoparathyroid

Compare *sitting height* with total height in children suspected of being dwarfs. Sitting height is most easily determined by having the child sit on a hard surface with the back against the wall and measuring from the top of the child's head to the surface. Normally, sitting height accounts for approximately 70% of total height at birth and decreases to about 60% at 2 years of age and to about 52% at 10 years of age. If the sitting height is greater than half the standing height, the patient has infantile stature; if the sitting height is approximately half the standing height, the patient has adult-type stature.

Children with sexual precocity and dwarfs with Morquio disease, mucopolysaccharidosis, or progeria attain adult body proportions early. Infantile stature persists or adult body proportions develop late in children with delayed adolescence, hypothyroidism, and some chondrodystrophies. Small children with normal body proportions for chronologic age may have genetically small stature, pituitary or primordial dwarfism, or gonadal dysgenesis. Children with sexual precocity grow rapidly before

Table 2-1. *Normal arm span minus height (cm)*

Age	Girls	Boys
Birth	−2.5	−2.5
10 yr	−1	0
12 yr	0	+2
15 yr	+1.2	+4.3

puberty and have shortened lower extremities when they are fully mature.

Abnormally *large growth* is rare and usually follows overfeeding or overeating, perhaps of psychologic origin. It also occurs in children with mental deficiency. True gigantism caused by excess growth hormone from an overactive pituitary is rare. Measure arm span in children with unusual growth patterns by stretching their arms parallel to the floor and holding the tape measure from fingertip to fingertip (Table 2-1). The span is more than 2 cm over height in children with Marfan syndrome, Klinefelter syndrome, homocystinuria, and congenital contractual arachnodactyly and is more than 2 cm less than height in children with bone or cartilage disorders or hypothyroidism.

WEIGHT

A child should be weighed routinely once a month for the first 6 months of life, once every 3 months for the next 6 months, twice a year for the next 3 years, and yearly thereafter. If you can not weigh a child because the child is holding the scale, say: "Hold your pants." The considerations of growth and development applied to height also apply to weight. Weight will often indicate that a problem exists sooner than will height alteration. The weight of the child should be compared with standard height–weight charts, and due allowances should be made for normal variations. Again, a single measurement tells little as compared with information obtained from serial measurements.

Acute *weight loss* indicates acute illness, dehydration, or malnutrition. Chronic weight loss suggests chronic disease states: These include improper food or feeding, diarrhea, cystic fibrosis or other gastrointestinal disturbances, emotional difficulties, respiratory difficulty during feeding, mental deficiency, and renal, cardiac, or connective tissue diseases.

Rapid *weight gain* may indicate overhydration or edema, but usually indicates overfeeding or overeating. A general overweight state (true obesity) is usually due to overfeeding or overeating—generally with a discernible psychologic background, but may be due to decreased activity, mental deficiency, or intracranial disorders. Rarely, endocrine disorders such as hyperadrenalism and hypothyroidism may be associated with obesity. In contrast to the obesity of overeating, these disorders are associated with retardation of linear growth. One estimation of body bulk, body mass index (BMI), is weight (in kilograms) divided by height (in square meters).

HEAD AND CHEST CIRCUMFERENCES

In infants aged less than 2 years, determine head and chest circumferences. Measure the head at its greatest circumference and the chest at the nipple line. Both measurements are needed for comparison.

At birth, the average head circumference of an infant is 34–37 cm; that of the chest is about 2 cm less. Head circumference usually approximates circumference of the chest until the child is aged 2 years, after which the chest continues to grow rapidly while head circumference increases only slightly. The significance of head and chest measurements is discussed in Chapter 4.

Body *asymmetry* may be noted. Such asymmetry is usually idiopathic but may be due to hemihypertrophy related to Wilms' tumor or other malignancies. Hemihypertrophy may also result from vascular anomalies, with increased perfusion and increased growth of the limb; it may also be due to hemiatrophy and associated with cerebral cortical injuries.

BLOOD PRESSURE

Measure blood pressure either before performing the examination or after the examination is complete. The patient should be relaxed and not crying. The proper cuff size is no less than half and no more than two thirds the length of the upper arm. Similar relative sizes are used for the thigh if leg pressures are taken. A larger cuff is difficult to apply and may give readings that are too low. A smaller cuff gives readings that are too high. The rubber bag inside the cuff must be long enough to encircle the arm completely. For very obese patients, apply the cuff to the forearm and auscultate at the wrist.

Compare the cuff to a balloon before applying it. An automated device uses a cuff, ultrasonic energy beamed from a transducer to a blood vessel or a recorder for systolic and diastolic pressures corresponding approximately to the first and fifth Korotkoff sounds. When using the manual device, allow the child to pump the cuff before it is wrapped. After wrapping the cuff snugly, place the manometer so that you and the child can see the "silver streak" of the mercury or the "clock" of the spring manometer. Place the bell stethoscope over the brachial artery.

Inflate the cuff higher than the expected systolic pressure and slowly deflate it. The wall of the collapsed vessel suddenly distends, producing the first Korotkoff sound—the systolic pressure. Further lowering is followed by a swishing sound, then a muffling—the fourth Korotkoff sound. Sound disappears at the fifth Korotkoff sound. Record systolic and diastolic pressures at the appearance and disappearance of Korotkoff sounds, recognizing that fifth phase recordings tend to underestimate diastolic pressure. Determining the fourth phase—muffling of the heart sounds—is less consistent. *Measure patients' blood pressure annually*, from the time the child is about 3 years of age.

If you cannot hear the Korotkoff sounds, you can make a rough estimate by applying the cuff in the usual manner, slowly deflating it, and palpating the radial, popliteal, or dorsalis pedis arteries. The first pulsation felt is about 10 mm below the true systolic pressure. If you cannot feel these arteries, the hand, wrist, and forearm (or toes, ankle, and leg) can be elevated and tightly wrapped to exclude blood up to the place where the cuff is applied. Then inflate the cuff to a level above the suspected blood pressure. Remove the wrappings. Slowly reduce the pressure in the cuff; the first flushing noted in the hand or foot is close to the systolic pressure.

If you fail in the first attempt at obtaining the blood pressure, remove the cuff before making another attempt, since even a deflated cuff may hurt or frighten the child. If you obtain an elevated blood pressure, repeat the measurement and measure the blood pressure in the other three extremities. In any patient suspected of having heart disease, measure the blood pressure in the four extremities.

Blood pressure at birth is about 60–90 mm Hg systolic and 20–60 mm Hg diastolic. Both pressures usually increase 2–3 mm per year of age; adult levels are reached near or soon after puberty (Fig. 2-1). Crying or apprehension may double these levels. Pulse pressure is normally 20–50 mm Hg throughout childhood. Systolic pressure in the arms may equal that in the legs in children until they are about 1 year of age. Thereafter the pressure in the legs should be about 10–30 mm Hg higher than that in the arms. The diastolic pressure should be almost equal in the arms and legs. If it is not, the cuff size is proper for the arms but too small for the legs. Very large differences in arm and leg systolic pressures (Hill's sign) suggest aortic insufficiency or coarctation of the aorta.

Elevated blood pressure values (both systolic and diastolic) may be noted. Blood pressure is usually elevated in one or both upper extremities of children with coarctation of the aorta or thoracic aortitis.

Hypertension

Kidney disease
  Pyelonephritis
  Acute glomerulonephritis
  Chronic glomerulonephritis
  Renal artery stenosis
  Nephrotic syndrome
  Renal tumors
  Renal calculi
Poisons
Bulbar poliomyelitis

Neuroblastoma
Familial dysautonomia
Increased intracranial pressure
Cushing disease
Pheochromocytoma
Neurofibromatosis
Hyperthyroid
Hypothyroid
Vitamin A or D poisoning
Spinal cord lesions

Children with scalenus anticus syndrome with cervical rib or with a coarctation of the aorta proximal to the left subclavian artery have *unequal blood pressures* in the arms. Some children with patent ductus arteriosus have unequal arm blood pressures.

Variable systolic pressures are *pulsus paradoxus*. Inflate and lower the pressure cuff several times. Irregular or fading beats occur with inspiration. The difference between the first faint sounds and repetitive crisp regular beats (the normal systolic difference with inspiration) is about 10 mm (see Chapter 5).

Elevated systolic pressure alone or with broadening of the pulse pressure is evident after exercise or excitement or in febrile states. It is usually associated with reduced diastolic

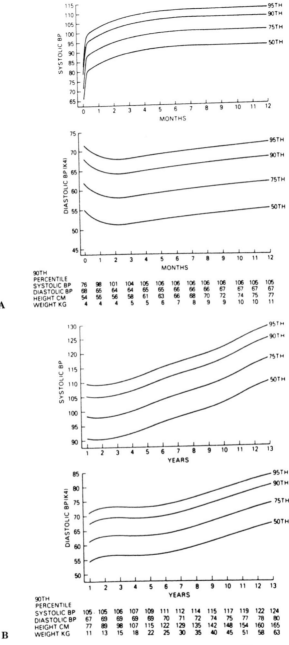

Figure 2-1. Age-specific percentiles of blood pressure (BP) measurements in girls from birth to 12 months of age; Korotkoff phase IV (K4) used for diastolic BP (**A**); girls from 1 to 13 years of age; K4 used for diastolic BP (**B**) (*courtesy American Academy of Pediatrics*).

A

90TH PERCENTILE

SYSTOLIC BP	76	98	101	104	105	106	106	106	106	106	106	105	105
DIASTOLIC BP	68	65	64	64	65	65	66	66	66	67	67	67	67
HEIGHT CM	54	55	56	58	61	63	66	68	70	72	74	75	77
WEIGHT KG	4	4	4	5	5	6	7	8	9	9	10	10	11

B

90TH PERCENTILE

SYSTOLIC BP	105	105	106	107	109	111	112	114	115	117	119	122	124
DIASTOLIC BP	67	69	69	69	69	70	71	72	74	75	77	78	80
HEIGHT CM	77	89	98	107	115	122	129	135	142	148	154	160	165
WEIGHT KG	11	13	15	18	22	25	30	35	40	45	51	58	63

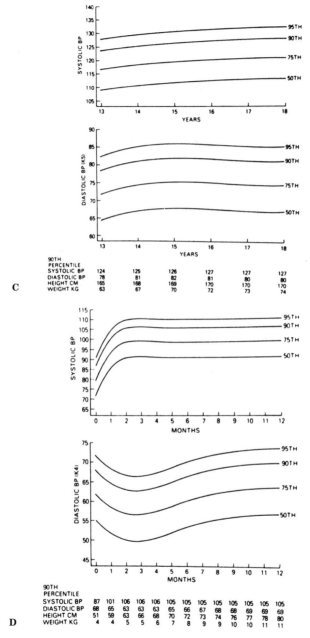

90TH PERCENTILE						
SYSTOLIC BP	124	125	126	127	127	127
DIASTOLIC BP	78	81	82	81	80	80
HEIGHT CM	165	168	169	170	170	170
WEIGHT KG	63	67	70	72	73	74

C

90TH PERCENTILE												
SYSTOLIC BP	87	101	106	106	106	105	105	105	105	105	105	105	105
DIASTOLIC BP	68	65	63	63	63	65	66	67	68	68	69	69	69
HEIGHT CM	51	59	63	66	68	70	72	73	74	76	77	78	80
WEIGHT KG	4	4	5	5	6	7	8	9	9	10	10	11	11

D

Figure 2-1. (*Continued*) Girls aged 13–18 years; Korotkoff phase V (K5) used for diastolic BP (**C**); boys from birth to 12 months of age; K4 used for diastolic BP (**D**).

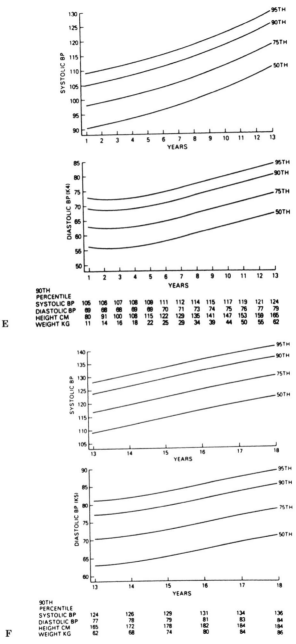

Figure 2-1. *(Continued)*   Boys aged 1–13 years; K4 used for diastolic BP (**E**); and boys aged 13–18 years; K5 used for diastolic BP (**F**).

pressure in children with patent ductus arteriosus, arteriovenous fistula, or aortic regurgitation.

Children with aortic or subaortic stenosis or with hypothyroidism have normal or elevated diastolic pressure with a low systolic pressure, and therefore a *narrow pulse pressure*. Children with aortic insufficiency or hyperthyroidism have widened or elevated pulse pressure.

Children with cardiac failure and children in a state of shock from causes such as heat exhaustion, circulatory collapse, blood loss, and adrenal insufficiency have *low blood pressure*. Newborns with trauma in the adrenal areas, children with meningococcemia and occasionally other septicemias, and children with chronic disease states or malnutrition have low blood pressure due to adrenal insufficiency. In children with Takayasu disease, arm blood pressure is low.

Orthostatic hypotension (a decrease in blood pressure of 15 mm Hg and/or an increase in pulse rate of 15 beats/min) occurs with a 20% loss of blood volume or some reflex vasodilatation or lack of vasoconstriction when an upright posture is assumed.

SKINFOLD MEASUREMENT

Place your thumb and forefinger of one hand just far enough apart so that you can pinch a full fold of the patient's skin and subcutaneous tissue firmly from the underlying tissue. Do not pick up muscle. Apply skinfold calipers just beneath your fin-

Table 2-2. *Approximate limits for midupper arm circumference and triceps skinfold*

Age	Midupper Arm Circumference Third to Fifth Percentile (cm)[a]	Triceps Skinfold 90th to 97th Percentile (mm)[b]	
		Boys	Girls
Newborn	9	10	10
3 mo	10	11	11
6 mo	11.5	12	12
9 mo	12	13	13
12 mo	13	14	14
2 yr	13	13	13
3 yr	13	13	13
4 yr	13.5	13	13
5 yr	13.5	13	13
6 yr	14	12	15
7 yr	14	13	16
8 yr	14.5	14	17
9 yr	15	14	18
10 yr	16	16	20
11 yr	16.5	17	21
12–16 yr	17–20	18–20	22–25

Modified from Zerfas A.J., Neumann C.G. Office assessment of nutritional status. *Pediatr Clin North Am* 1977; 24:253.

[a] A lower value suggests undernutrition.

[b] A higher value suggests obesity.

gers. Calipers should apply a constant pressure of about 10 g/mm^2. Make measurements at the back of the upper arms over the triceps midway between the elbow and tip of the acromial process. Measure midupper arm circumference with a flexible tape. Measurements of skinfold help in identifying obesity; those of circumference help in identifying and following malnutrition as an indication of body composition. Representative values are shown in Table 2-2. In adolescents, the desirable sum of skinfold measurements of triceps and calf is 10–30 mm.

General Appearance, Skin, and Lymph Nodes

The future of a civilization may be judged by how it cares for its young.

Senator Daniel Patrick Moynihan

The general appearance of a child may reveal much more than subtle physical findings. On first seeing the child, sit down and slowly observe the child. Does the child look well or ill? Does the child appear comfortable or uncomfortable, and if uncomfortable, in what way? Is the breathing easy or difficult? Is the child in any type of physical or emotional distress? Is the child's appearance alert or lethargic? Is the child clean or dirty? Is the child's attitude cooperative or belligerent? Does the child have any gross abnormalities or anomalies? Is the child fat or thin or tall or short? Does the child appear to be malnourished? Is the child apprehensive and, if so, is the apprehension due to new surroundings, to the parents, to the examiner, or to the disease? Is the child interested in the new instruments presented by the physician? Does the child obey the mother and the physician or fight them? If the child obeys, is the obedience due to fear? Is the child excited or calm? Does the child twitch and fidget? In essence, is the child similar to peers or different from them, and if different, in what way?

When you record the child's general features, describe the facies (facial expression and appearance) and use terms such as chronically ill, alert, comatose, lethargic, dull, responsive, hostile, and cooperative. These descriptive terms should start you on the road to proper diagnosis. Dirt, feces, or other signs of neglect alert you to possible child abuse. Also note the interaction between the patient and the parents throughout the examination. Pediatricians are fortunate because their patients, unlike adults, rarely dissimulate. Regardless of what the mother says about the patient, experienced pediatricians know that a child who does not look ill is usually not acutely ill and that a child who looks ill is usually acutely or chronically ill.

During the course of each examination, the child should be completely undressed. With infants, it is easiest to have the mother completely undress the child before the examination. In older children, respect shyness and any reticence and examine them by removing and replacing articles of their clothing as each portion of examination is completed.

If a patient is acutely ill, try to determine the system involved and the degree of distress. For example, flaring nostrils indicate a problem in the respiratory or cardiac system, and delirium, coma, or convulsions indicate a problem in the central nervous system (CNS). Note the nature of the cry of the child. A strong, loud cry may indicate that the child is in pain, is frightened, or simply wishes to cry. Even a strong cry is helpful in diagnosis because it usually indicates that the child is not weak or debilitated. In contrast, a weak cry may indicate that the child is weak, debilitated, or gravely ill. A screeching, high-pitched cry may indicate that the child has increased intracranial pressure or other CNS lesions. In infants, a hoarse, low-pitched cry may be normal or may indicate laryngeal abnormalities, tetany, or cretinism.

Normal newborns may be asleep or crying, but older children are responsive during examinations. A child who smiles, chats, and laughs is usually well or only moderately ill. A child who cries constantly may be more seriously ill.

A child who lies quietly with few movements and stares into space may be gravely ill or may have been abused. A child with paradoxical hyperirritability may lie quietly on the examining table only to scream when picked up by the mother. This is a valuable sign, since most children are calmed when picked up, and may indicate a serious disturbance in the CNS system (particularly meningitis), pain in motion (which occurs in scurvy, fracture, cortical hyperostosis, and acrodynia), or a serious disturbance in response to painful stimuli.

A child with acute illness may have parched skin and tongue, sunken dry eyes, a weak cry, and exhausted and lethargic behavior, as may children with dehydration or acute or chronic malnutrition. In patients with febrile states, the eyes may appear bright and apprehensive.

A child in pain may cry, wince, double up, rub the painful part, or display general fretfulness and other signs of discomfort. Older children can indicate the site and sometimes the cause of the pain. Painful facies may be modified in a few disease states. For example, a child with peritonitis lies ominously still, the nares flare, and respiration is entirely thoracic and very shallow. With intussusception, the child lies very still one moment and claws, twists, and screams the next moment. Watch the face of the child for apprehension as you examine other parts of the body. Palpating over a tender abdomen may elicit a grimace in a stoic child even as the child says: "It doesn't hurt." A grimace or a change in cry of the child as you palpate over the bladder or in the costovertebral angle may be a true sign of renal disease.

A dyspneic child demonstrates very rapid respiration, flaring of the nares, and possibly some cyanosis about the lips. The child may be irritable and hyperactive, possibly apprehensive, and may appear to be fighting for air. In a child with carbon dioxide retention, confusion, stupor, and finally shock may be added to these signs.

The facies of a child with nasal obstruction is characterized by mouth breathing, an open mouth, narrow pinched nose, high palate, dull appearance, and nasal voice; the sternum may be sunken. Children with hypertrophied adenoids or chronic sinusitis may exhibit this type of facies, with swelling over the cheeks.

The facies of a developmentally delayed child is sometimes diagnostic. The eyes are dull, the face is blank, and the child is unresponsive. Developmental delay in children may be due to hereditary factors, maternal infections (especially in the first trimester of pregnancy), congenital anomalies of the brain, or degenerative neurologic disorders. It is commonly due to cerebral injury, sequelae of infections, or hypoxic ischemic encephalopathy and is frequently accompanied by other signs of cerebral palsy. However, delay must not be assumed in all children who have a dull expression. Children who are deaf or blind or who have specific language difficulties and children with prolonged illness or psychologic difficulties may have a similar facies, one easily mistaken for mental deficiency.

Note the *position* the child assumes during the examination. Abnormal, resistant, or persistent positioning may be caused by muscular, neurologic, or emotional disorders. For example, a child with torticollis or cerebellar disease may lean the head toward the affected side, a child with appendicitis or other painful intraabdominal conditions may lie on the affected side with the leg of that side flexed at the hip and knee, and a child with unilateral labyrinthitis may insist on lying only on the affected side.

Likewise, voluntary or involuntary *movement* or *lack of movement* may direct attention to a particular system. For example, a brain-injured child with spastic paresis may keep the arm flexed at the elbow, and the wrist and fingers may be held stiffly in flexion. With extensive cerebral involvement, the child may be entirely in extensor spasticity; with cerebellar involvement, the child may be ataxic; and with basal ganglia involvement, the child may be athetoid and grimacing. Stereotaxic movements may suggest neurologic disorders.

Estimate the state of nutrition. Acute malnutrition manifests as loss of weight and skin turgor. Chronic malnutrition may be evident. Overnutrition is recognized as obesity and unusual weight gain. (Causes of weight loss and gain are discussed in Chapter 2.)

Signs of Chronic Malnutrition

Low weight	Bony prominences
Protuberant abdomen	Flat buttocks
Muscle wasting	Poor muscle tone
Slow response to stimuli	Prominent sucking pads in cheeks

Note Development. Assess the patient's response to you and the surroundings, noting speech, action, and crying, and make a rapid estimate of mental development. Gross deviations from normal are apparent at a glance if the child appears dull or does not respond. Estimate gross physical development for the age and confirm by direct measurement.

Speech is one of the developmental signs least dependent on motor ability and should be noted in very young children. A 3-month-old infant may "coo" and a 7-month-old infant may say "ma-ma" and "da-da". A few more words are added at 1 year of age, and short sentences are added at 2 years of age. A 3-year-old child, even if not frightened, may stutter or stammer (see Appendix C). A child's failure to develop speech may be due to motor incoordination of the speech muscles but is commonly due to a lack of desire to speak because of adequate communication by other means. Such children respond to simple commands readily. Other causes of failure to speak include lack of stimulus by parents or environment, deafness, mental retardation, histidinemia, or psychologic disturbances. Severe dysarthria is a sign of spastic quadriplegia.

You can keep a convenient record of your patients' development by using the Denver Developmental Screening Test (Appendix B).

Markedly advanced motor signs such as early rolling over, early head control with poor feeding, and decreased spontaneous muscle movements suggest spastic cerebral palsy.

ODOR

Some infants and children will have distinct body *odors*. A few of these odors are associated with diseases (Table 3-1).

SKIN

Although *observation* of the skin is essential to dermatologic diagnosis, do not neglect *palpation* of skin lesions. Examine the skin as a whole or examine each underlying part. Regardless of the method you adopt, note the condition of the skin of the entire body each time you examine the patient. If skin lesions are found, note their distribution, *color*, and character.

Normal pigmentation is caused by melanin in the skin; depigmented areas are termed *vitiligo*. Small depigmented patches may be caused by tinea versicolor, pityriasis alba or rosea, or dermatophytosis. When they are accompanied by structural or developmental defects, chromosome abnormalities may be present. Unpigmented streaks covering large areas of the body may represent hypomelanosis of Ito, frequently associated with CNS abnormalities. In children, vitiligo in small leaf-shaped patches which may fluoresce may be the first sign of tuberous sclerosis or

Table 3-1. *Odors of patient or urine*

Odors	Disease
Musty or "mousy"	Phenylketonuria, diphtheria
Maple syrup	Maple syrup urine disease
Sweaty sock	Isovaleric or glutaric II acidemia
Brewery, fishy	Methionine metabolism, oasthouse
Garlic	Arsenic, thallium, parathion, or phosphorus poisoning, tellurium, selenium, DMSO
Bitter almond	Cyanide poisoning
"Tom-cat" urine	3-methylcrotonyl CoA carboxylase (biotin) deficiency
Onion	Selenium poisoning
Acetone	Isopropyl alcohol, methanol poisoning, acidosis
Wintergreen	Methyl salicylate poisoning
Violets	Turpentine poisoning
Pear	Chloral hydrate poisoning
Shoe polish	Nitrobenzene poisoning
Coal gas	Carbon monoxide poisoning
Cabbage	Tyrosinosis
Stench	Foreign body in nose, vagina, ear
Fish (spoiled)	Trimethylaminuria
Fish	Kidney failure
Fresh brown bread	Typhoid
Urine	Uremia

DMSO, dimethyl sulfoxide.

other neuroectodermal disease. Generalized lack of pigmentation occurs in albinism, an inborn error of tyrosine metabolism, and in the Chédiak-Steinbrinck-Higashi syndrome.

Localized areas of increased pigmentation (nevi) are common. Note the size and color and presence of hair. Various shades of red nevi are usually of vascular origin (*hemangiomas*). Small vascular nevi with small radiating vessels caused by capillary dilation may be easily compressed. Because of their appearance, they are termed *spider nevi* or *spider angiomas*. A few may be present on the arms or hands or high on the face of normal children. In patients with cirrhosis or hepatitis, such nevi are larger and more common on the trunk.

Port-wine stains are pink to purple with irregular borders. Where they involve the trigeminal nerve, they may cause eye and brain abnormalities (Sturge-Weber syndrome). When associated with the venous system, they cause hypertrophy of the limb (Klippel-Trenaunay-Weber syndrome). Multiple hemangiomas may cause skeletal abnormalities (Maffuci syndrome or Gorham disease); others cause intestinal bleeding (blue rubber bleb syndrome). Any hemangioma can be associated with petechiae or bleeding because of trapping of platelets (Kasabach-Merritt syndrome).

Yellow, brown, or black nevi are usually local melanin deposits. Nevi over the lower spine may overlie spina bifida occulta or tethering of the cord. Large coarse nevi may represent the epidermal nevus syndrome, which is associated with congenital anomalies. Linear or circular sebaceous or waxy nevi and giant pigmented nevi over the buttocks may become malignant.

Multiple small pigmented spots are termed *freckles*. Multiple freckles in the axillary region are common in patients with neurofibromatosis. Multiple freckles are apparent in children with either the multiple lentigenes or Bannayan-Riley-Ruvacalba syndrome.

Increased dark pigmentation, especially over the exposed areas, is most frequently due to sun or windburn.

Increased Pigment

Addison disease
Hemosiderosis
Hypothyroidism
Argyria
Pellagra
Lupus erythematosus

A pellagralike symmetric browning of the dorsal aspects of the hands on exposure to sunlight may be associated with cerebellar ataxia in Hartnup syndrome, a metabolic defect. *Photosensitivity* results from use of some drugs and is also characteristic of errors in porphyrin metabolism.

Children with polyostotic fibrous dysplasia have light-brown asymmetric pigmented areas. Darker patches (*café au lait* spots) are evident in patients with neurofibromatosis and are a diagnostic sign of the disorder in children aged less than 5 years, especially if more than five are apparent and are more than 1 cm long. Fibromas along the course of a nerve are another sign of neurofibromatosis.

Large, flat, black or blue-black areas are frequently noted over the sacrum and buttocks. They are termed *mongolian spots* and have no pathologic significance. Bluish-black, soft, verrucous symmetric areas of the axillae, neck, and knuckles are characteristic of acanthosis nigricans and are sometimes associated with malignancies, genetic abnormalities, drug use, and endocrine diseases.

Look for *cyanosis* and jaundice. Cyanosis is a bluish discoloration of a normally pink area and is most easily detected in the nail beds or in the mucous membranes of the mouth. It occurs when a minimum of 5 g/dL reduced hemoglobin is present, regardless of the total level of hemoglobin. Therefore, cyanosis develops less easily in an anemic child, more easily in a child with polycythemia, and not at all in a child with anemia with a hemoglobin content less than 5 g/dL. Visible cyanosis is not a good estimate of the degree of oxygen unsaturation except when the total amount of hemoglobin is 12–15 g/dL or more.

Central cyanosis is always a cause for concern because of its association with pulmonary, cardiovascular, central nervous system, and hematologic disorders.

Central Cyanosis

Pulmonary Disease
Atelectasis
Pneumonia
Cystic fibrosis
Lung anomalies

Cyanotic Congenital Heart Disease
Transposition
Tetralogy of Fallot
Tricuspid atresia
Anomalous venous return
Truncus
Pulmonary atresia
Congestive heart failure

To recognize central cyanosis, do not look at the patient's nail beds or around the mouth. Look at the tongue. With peripheral cyanosis, the tongue is pink; with central cyanosis, the tongue is blue. Peripheral cyanosis is caused by excessive removal of oxygen from blood at the tissue level and is usually caused by slowing of blood through the capillary bed due to hypothermia, local venous obstruction, vasomotor instability, and occasionally to shock with sepsis or congestive heart failure.

Other causes of cyanosis include obstruction of the respiratory tract, prolonged crying, temper tantrums with breath-holding, convulsive states, acrocyanosis, and shock. Cyanosis may occur with as little as 1–2 g/dL abnormal hemoglobin as a result of poisoning, as in methemoglobinemia and sulfhemoglobinemia.

Compare the patient's upper and lower extremities with respect to cyanosis. The lower extremities may be more cyanotic than the upper extremities in patients with coarctation of the aorta or in patients with pulmonary hypertension with patent ductus arteriosus. The lower extremities may be less cyanotic than the upper extremities in children with transposition of the great vessels with patent ductus. Acrocyanosis not caused by heart or lung disease occurs with vasospasm (Raynaud's phenomenon); children with Kawasaki disease have a blue discoloration of the feet of unknown cause.

Veins are normally apparent through the thin skin of many children. Distended veins in the arms and legs are usually due to dependent position. Dilated veins elsewhere may be due to cardiac decompensation or local venous obstruction and are also evident in children with cyanosis. *Collateral arterial circulation* is rare in children.

Determine *direction of blood flow* if fistula, collateral circulation, or obstruction is suspected. First, empty the vessel by placing two fingers together and then pushing one finger along the course of the vessel for 1–2 inches. If the vessel fills before pressure is released, collateral circulation is present. Then release pressure of one finger. If the vessel fills after release of pressure, blood flows from the area of pressure release toward the area where pressure is still being applied. If the vessel does not fill, replace the first finger, release the second, and similarly observe the direction of blood flow. If the vessel still does not fill, poor circulation in the area is suggested.

The area over a vein may be tender with infection in the vein (*thrombophlebitis*). When thrombophlebitis becomes extensive and causes obstruction to blood flow, the veins may become tortuous, dilated, and easily palpable. Phlebitis of the deep veins of the legs can be elicited by forcibly flexing the foot and noting pain in the calf (Homan sign). In children, phlebitis usually results from infection spreading from an area near the vein or from embolism or thrombosis.

Jaundice can be manifest as various shades of yellow or green and is best observed by examining the patient's sclera, skin, or mucous membranes in daylight; it may be missed entirely in artificial light. It occurs in newborns when the total serum bilirubin is more than 5 mg/dL and is evident in older children when total bilirubin is more than 2 mg/dL. It is caused by cellular or obstructive liver disease or hemolysis.

Jaundice

Hepatitis
Poisons
Leptospirosis
Infectious mononucleosis
Hemolysis
Biliary obstruction
Choledochal cyst

In infections, especially pneumonia and congenital syphilis, jaundice may also appear anywhere in the body. Jaundice occurs in cholestasis and in prolonged parenteral alimentation. It is rarely caused by bile duct stones in childhood, although such stones sometimes occur after episodes of hemolysis. Pruritis is common in jaundice.

A pale, yellow-orange tint of the skin may be due to carotenemia and is most prominent over the palms, soles, and nasolabial folds. Carotenemia is due to excess carotene ingestion but may be an early sign of hypothyroidism. It occasionally occurs in diabetic children. Children with severe hemolytic anemias have a peculiar yellowness of the skin unrelated to jaundice.

Note *pallor* or paleness. In darkly pigmented children, it is most easily detected in the nail beds, conjunctivas, oral mucosa, or tongue, which are normally reddish-pink. Pallor should never be considered an accurate estimate of hemoglobin concentration. It is usually a normal complexion characteristic or sign of indoor living, but it may indicate anemia, chronic disease, edema, or shock. *Plethora*, due to polycythemia, is usually not easily detected in children.

Generalized *erythematous* rashes are common in children.

Erythematous Rashes

Rubeola	Toxic shock
Rubella	Toxic epidermal neurolysis
Roseola	Staphylococcal scalded skin
Parvovirus	Kawasaki disease
Scarlatina	Drug reaction

Erythematous lesions of varying types appearing simultaneously, with peripheral spreading and central clearing, are characteristic of erythema multiforme. Red patches that expand centrifugally are erythema chronicum migrans, characteristic of Lyme disease. If these lesions are 2–4 cm in diameter and are painful, tender, and nodular (especially along the shins), they are erythema nodosum. The lesions may be skin manifestations of systemic diseases.

Erythema Nodosum

Systemic	**Drugs**
Rheumatic fever	Sulfonamides
Streptococcosis	Oral contraceptives
Tuberculosis	Aspartame
Sarcoid	Bromides
Inflammatory bowel disease	Iodides
Behçet's syndrome	
Rheumatoid arthritis	**Other Infections**
Stevens-Johnson syndrome	Leprosy
Lupus erythematosus	Salmonellosis
Vasculitis	Yersiniosis
	Chlamydiae
	Cat-scratch fever
	Fungi

Erythema nodosum is more common in girls, particularly at puberty, than in boys. Similar single lesions on the hands, feet, knees, or buttocks, usually a raised circle with normal skin inside and outside the erythematous area, may be characteristic of granuloma annulare, which may be due to sensitivity to penicillin or other agents. Nontender erythematous patches on the palms and soles (Janeway lesions) occur in children with acute bacterial endocarditis. Serpiginous erythematous "lines" suggest cutaneous larva migrans.

A *fleeting*, purplish erythematous rash lasting a few minutes to a few hours and recurring at short intervals may be observed in children with rheumatoid arthritis. Erythema that is *annular* or circinate, 1–2 cm in diameter, serpiginous, and flat with erythematous margins surrounding intact skin over the arms, trunk, and legs but not on the face is erythema marginatum. It is characteristic of rheumatic fever. The rash may change from hour to hour.

Localized, painful, hot, erythematous, indurated areas with raised borders are characteristic of erysipelas. Erysipelas is usually caused by streptococcal infection of the skin and is accompanied by high fever. Localized, painful, hot, erythematous, indurated areas lacking raised borders are characteristic of cellulitis. A blue discoloration in the center, particularly in children aged less than 3 years, frequently indicates infection due to *Haemophilus influenzae*. Lesions of similar appearance, particularly around the face, occur with cold injury and frostbite (cold panniculitis). Cellulitis is due to infection in the subcutaneous tissues and may overlie areas of osteomyelitis of bone or thrombophlebitis.

The most common erythematous eruptions, however, are of varying extent and may be due to almost any type of irritation. In the diaper area, erythema is an early form of diaper rash—a type of contact dermatitis—and also occurs in Kawasaki disease. Wind, sun, wool, or clothing may cause erythema of the face or other exposed parts. Excoriation of the convex surfaces of the buttocks is usually due to chafing or excessive moisture. The region around the anus is usually excoriated after loose stools, whereas excoriation around the mucocutaneous area may be due to congenital syphilis. Excoriation of opposing surfaces, especially in the creases of the neck or axillae, is intertrigo and may be due to seborrheic dermatitis or to moisture, with maceration of the skin with constant irritation. In monilia infection, the excoriations are red and scaly and sharply outlined.

Pruritus

Common infections	Skin irritants
Jaundice	Drugs
Allergies	Lymphoma
Iron deficiency	Diabetes
Uremia	

Diffuse redness of the hands and feet, especially if associated with severe pain, suggests a diagnosis of acrodynia, although boric acid poisoning may cause similar signs. Intermittent pallor or cyanosis of the fingers and toes may be an early sign of Raynaud phenomenon. This condition is usually painless, may be aggravated by cold or emotion, and is due to arteriolar spasm with sympathetic nervous system overactivity. Faint erythematous streaks, especially near sites of infection or injury, which follow the course of lymphatics, are inflamed superficial lymph vessels and indicate lymphangitis. Children with fifth disease (erythema infectiosum) caused by parvovirus exhibit bright confluent warm, tender erythema of the cheeks, as though the face had been slapped, that blanches on pressure and fades in 1–4 days. Intense facial redness with pruritus occurs with rifampin toxicity. Any irritant may cause pruritis.

Discrete nonraised lesions are termed *macules*. The rapid appearance of many macules is characteristic of the exanthemata: measles, German measles, scarlet fever, roseola infantum, and typhoid fever. Distinguishing the exanthemata from drug rashes is sometimes difficult, especially when the macules are caused by penicillin or atropine. Similar eruptions may be observed in children with rickettsial diseases or infectious mononucleosis and other viral diseases, particularly the echovirus and coxsackievirus groups and human immunodeficiency virus. Similar eruptions are apparent in fourth disease (Dukes' disease or mild scarlatina) and in erythema infectiosum. A German-measles-like rash was formerly evident 7–10 days after smallpox vaccination.

Firm skin and subcutaneous elevations with discoloration are *papules*. Papules may occur with any of the exanthemata after the macular stage and may also occur after any condition that causes the appearance of macules. Small gray or white papules are apparent in sarcoid. Red, circular, nonhemorrhagic areas 1–2 cm in diameter over the chest, thighs, or elsewhere on the body evidencing scratch marks may be due to ringworm. A large, purplish, maculopapular, scaly, oval area surrounded by smaller, similar lesions is characteristic of pityriasis rosea. Sharply raised, red, scaly areas over the elbows and knees are characteristic of psoriasis. Erythematous papules over the finger joints suggest dermatomyositis.

Skin elevations containing serous fluid are *vesicles* or blisters. In chickenpox, lesions itch, are in varied stages, and may cover the body, including the axilla and head. In contrast to the other vesicular diseases, in herpes zoster, pain, if present, precedes the appearance of vesicles.

Important Childhood Vesicular Lesions

Chicken pox: appear in crops
Herpes simplex: fever blisters near mouth
Herpes zoster: along nerves
Insect bites: exposed areas
Ivy or other poisons: exposed areas
Molluscum: umbilicated
Rickettsial pox: on top of maculopapules

Larger vesicles are termed *blebs* or *bullae*.

Bullae

Burns (? abuse)
Scarlet fever (palms, soles)
Congenital syphilis (palms, soles)
Sunburn, ivy, oak poisoning
Summer eruption (hydroa estivale)
Porphyria (photosensitive)
Epidermolysis bullosa (irritation)
Pemphigoid
Dermatitis herpetiformis

Larger vesicles are termed *blebs* or *bullae*. They occur in children with the bullous form of erythema multiforme or immune-deficient diseases. Bullae at birth followed by zebralike pigmentation are characteristic of incontinentia pigmenti or epidermolytic hyperkeratosis, which are congenital malformations of the ectoderm. Children with diarrhea who have acrodermatitis enteropathica manifest bullae of the ends of the fingers; the bullae are responsive to zinc.

Tender skin with erythema followed by bullae that may rub off is Nikolsky sign.

Nikolsky Sign

Toxic epidermal necrolysis (TEN): drugs
Staph-scalded skin syndrome (SSSS): staphylococcus
Stevens-Johnson syndrome (SJS): drugs, mucosa
Toxic shock syndrome: hands, feet
Kawasaki disease: hands, feet

Skin elevations containing purulent fluid are *pustules*. Pustules are usually due to bacterial infection or skin abscesses. Pustules may also be evident after any of the states causing vesicles: in adolescents with acne, on the finger in herpes (herpetic whitlow), or after poisoning, such as with iodine. Groups of pustules due to staphylococci or streptococci are known as *impetigo*. Deeper infections, termed *ecthyma*, probably start as impetigo. Larger abscesses of the hair follicles or sebaceous glands are *furuncles* or *carbuncles*. Small straight lines or *burrows* associated with papules, vesicles, or pustules may be scabies, which are due to the itch mite. These lesions may appear anywhere on the body of the child (in contrast to the more localized distribution on the hands and groin of the adult) and are usually accompanied by signs of itching.

Necrotic areas of the superficial and deep layers of the skin, skin *ulcers*, are common in adults with vascular insufficiency. They occasionally occur on the legs of children with sickle cell anemia. Ulceration may occur after skin has been destroyed by burns or trauma or, as a result of hypersensitivity, after subcutaneous injection of antigens.

Petechiae are small, reddish-purple spots in the superficial layers of the skin. If palpable, they frequently indicate severe systemic disease caused by bacterial emboli or vasculitis, as occurs in meningococcemia, rickettsial diseases, leptospirosis, other overwhelming systemic infections or bacterial endocarditis, disseminated intravascular coagulation (DIC), and juvenile rheumatoid arthritis. Petechiae are not palpable in conditions in which platelets are inadequate or defective, as in thrombocytopenic or nonthrombocytopenic purpura, or when capillary permeability is increased, as in scurvy or leukemia. More frequently, they may be caused by injury or by increased capillary pressure due to severe coughing (especially pertussis), allergies in which the cause is unknown, or direct trauma. Paler red or pink areas that measure 0.5 mm may be petechiae or *rose spots*, characteristic of typhoid fever or other *Salmonella* infections.

Ecchymoses, which are evidence of blood under the skin, are usually due to bruising or other injury, but they may be a sign of increased bleeding tendency such as occurs in hemophilia, leukemia, or the purpuras. Purple-red bruises that are fresh, dark blue, or brown are 1–4 days old; greenish-yellow bruises are about 5–7 days old, and yellow bruises are more than 1 week old and healing. Multiple hematomas may indicate child abuse; such hematomas found in the genitalia may indicate sexual abuse.

Localized areas of swelling and scratch marks are characteristic of *hives* (urticaria or wheals), papular urticaria, insect bites, scabies, and ivy and sumac poisoning. Localized small swellings or excrescences without scratch marks may be warts. Scratch marks with ulcers, ecchymoses, itching, and other skin lesions may be due to neurodermatitis or may be self-inflicted factitial dermatitis.

Increased sensitivity to skin pressure manifested by wheals or bright red lines is characteristic of *dermatographia*, a form of urticaria. Dermatographia is easily produced by lightly scratching the skin with your nail and is most easily noted over the back or upper chest. Especially persistent dermatographia (*tache cérébrale*) is a sign of CNS irritation particularly apparent in patients with tuberculous meningitis. Large wheal formation after stroking may be a sign of generalized mast cell disease (urticaria pigmentosa) and is common in comatose patients who have taken an overdose of depressant agents.

Subcutaneous nodules are usually due to absorbing or calcifying hematomas (see list below), sterile abscesses, or poorly absorbed injections.

Cutaneous Calcification (Calcinosis Cutis)

Scleroderma	Dermatomyositis
Hyperparathyroidism	Hypervitaminosis D
Sarcoid	Excess milk ingestion
Osteomyelitis	Uremia
Leukemia	Metastatic carcinoma

Nodules over the extensor surfaces of the joints or near the occipital protuberances may aid in the diagnosis of rheumatic fever, rheumatoid arthritis, lupus erythematosus, and granuloma annulare. They may be tender. Red tender nodules on the fingertips, thumbs, or footpads (Osler nodes) are pathognomonic of subacute bacterial endocarditis. Subcutaneous nodules (blueberry muffin spots) are a characteristic of neuroblastoma.

Small yellow or orange plaques (*xanthomas*) on the skin, particularly about the nasal bridge, are usually due to local accumulations of fatty substance. Xanthomas may occur as isolated findings, particularly in infancy, or may be a manifestation of any condition causing hyperlipemia, hypercholesterolemia, or hypertriglyceridemia. The reticuloendothelioses may also cause xanthomas. Pigmented or depigmented xanthomalike lesions may be adenoma sebaceum, characteristic of tuberous sclerosis.

Cysts may be felt under the skin as superficial masses with fluid. They are usually nontender and may transilluminate light. A cyst over the dorsum of the hand or wrist is most commonly a ganglion—a degenerated cyst of the tendon sheath. Tumors of the skin may be firm or soft and are usually lipomas or fibromas. *Atrophic* areas of the skin may result from injury or, in diabetic patients with diabetes, from use of insulin.

Feel the skin. The texture may be rough, as is common in children during the winter, especially after contact with wool or soap. In children with hyperkeratosis, the skin may be rough due to vitamin A deficiency, hypothyroidism, or hypoparathyroidism. Rough dry skin, especially over the legs, may be a manifestation of ichthyosis. Thickening of the skin in the flexor folds of the elbows and knees is characteristic of chronic eczema. The skin also hardens and thickens in sclerema, scleredema, scleroderma, and dermatomyositis.

Yellow, dirty scaling beginning on the scalp is termed *cradle cap*. Scaling beginning on the scalp and proceeding down the face and body, associated with erythema, is a self-limited form of exfoliative seborrheic dermatitis (Leiner disease), which appears in the first 3 months of life. Scaling that begins on the cheeks and spreads to the forehead, scalp, posterior of the ears, and down the body is characteristic of infantile eczema, which begins about the second month of life and lasts 1–2 years. Eczema may occur in conditions of immunologic deficiency or in some metabolic diseases. Scaling in the diaper area, sometimes associated with vesiculation and infection, may occur with diaper rash. Scaling with plaques or vesicles on the plantar surface of the foot may occur with psoriasis, allergic contact dermatitis, or juvenile plantar dermatosis.

Skin Scaling

Seborrhea	
Eczema	**Dietary Deficiency**
Histiocytosis	Zinc
Contact dermatitis	Biotin
Ringworm	Selenium
Epidermophytoses	Essential
Dyshydrosis	Fatty acids
Posterythematous eruptious	
Congenital syphilis	
Kawasaki disease	

Subcutaneous emphysema is felt as a crackling or crepitant sensation under the skin. It is most commonly associated with pneumothorax, pneumomediastinum, and gas gangrene. A similar sensation is evident if one palpates an area over a bone fracture.

Striae are usually pale white or pink lines occurring in localized areas that are growing rapidly, such as the lower abdomen or thighs of an obese child. They usually occur after overeating or during the growth spurt, but striking purple striae may indicate the presence of Cushing syndrome. Scars are red or white lines and are evidence of previous injury or operation. Scars become elevated when keloid formation occurs.

Estimate the degree of sweating. In infants sweating normally begins after the first month of life. Sweating, especially in children aged less than 1 year, may be profuse and is usually caused by exercise, crying, an overly warm atmosphere, or eating. Profuse sweating, however, may be caused by fever, hypoglycemia, hyperthyroidism, congenital heart disease, hypocalcemia, acrodynia,

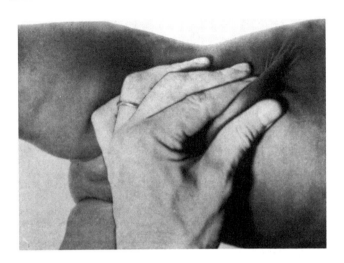

Figure 3-1. Subcutaneous turgor or elasticity. It is best demonstrated by grasping the skin and subcutaneous tissue over the abdomen and allowing it to fall back in place.

pneumothorax, cystic fibrosis, or fear. Night sweats may be caused by sleep apnea or spinal cord injuries. Dry skin (anhidrosis) is also normal but may be a sign of dehydration, coma, atropine poisoning, hypothyroidism, eczema, or ectodermal dysplasia.

Feel the skin for tissue turgor, elasticity, and edema. Tissue *turgor* is determined by pinching the skin, squeezing out the blood, and watching color change. Slow return of color denotes decreased turgor, a sign of decreased subcutaneous tissue or shock. Estimate the *capillary refill time* (return of color), which normally is less than 2 seconds. Color returns in 2–3 seconds with 50–90 mL/kg fluid depletion and in more than 3 seconds with more than 100 mL/kg, which constitutes medical shock. This test is inaccurate if heart failure or hypertonic dehydration is present. Tissue *elasticity* is best determined by grasping 1 or 2 inches of the patient's skin and subcutaneous tissues over the abdominal wall between the thumb and index finger, squeezing, and allowing the skin to fall back in place (Fig. 3-1). It is an estimate of status of hydration and nutrition. Normally, the skin appears smooth and firm and, when grasped as described, quickly falls back in place without residual marks. The skin remains suspended and creased for a few seconds in children with poor elasticity.

The tissues feel plastic and doughy in children with chronic wasting disease, peritonitis, or hyperelectrolytemia with dehydration. Little subcutaneous tissue will be felt in malnourished children. The skin will remain suspended and in folds in dehydrated patients. This may not occur in obese infants; if dehydration is suspected in them, other signs should be sought. Poor tissue turgor may be apparent in a normal infant a few days old, especially in premature infants, but they rapidly add fat and subcutaneous tissue so that turgor is normal by body weight of 2000 gm or more.

The skin normally feels firm, especially over the legs. Calluses occur frequently on the hands or feet following constant irritation. Thickening over the knuckles (knuckle pads) may be due to induced vomiting in patients with bulimia nervosa. The skin feels thin and loosely filled in children with chronic diseases, malnutrition, and rickets. It may feel very soft and flabby in children with flaccid paralyses and in children with muscle diseases such as myasthenia gravis or amyotonia congenita, as well as in children with developmental delay. The skin may be soft and mushy in children with Down syndrome. It may feel hard and thickened in children with hypothyroidism, whether the condition is congenital or acquired. Other unusual texture is described in Chapter 9.

The skin may be tender to touch. This may indicate that the child is irritable or has CNS disease or another systemic illness. Referred pain is due particularly to intraabdominal disease. Pain elicited by light pressure is more likely due to cellulitis and deeper pressure to bone or joint infections. Painful skin over the right lower abdominal wall may signify acute appendicitis. Skin tenderness is also noted in polyneuritis, and children with ruptured spleen display tenderness over the left shoulder. Tenderness may be due to a cryptic foreign body such as a splinter. Transilluminate (particularly the fingers or toes) to help localize the object.

Impressions in the skin that remain for several seconds following finger pressure occur in patients with pitting *edema*. Edema is the presence of an abnormal amount of extracellular fluid and is caused by an increase in hydrostatic pressure, increased capillary permeability, decreased oncotic pressure, increased retention of sodium or other electrolytes, mechanical obstruction of the lymphatic channels, lymphedema, or decreased excretion of water. Puffy-appearing areas on the body that do not pit or leave marks after pressure or pinching are termed *nonpitting edema*. For example, cretins manifest puffy skin with no pitting. Scleredema, a rare connective tissue disease, is a firm nonpitting edema affecting face, neck, scalp, conjunctivae, thorax, and occasionally the arms and legs but not the feet.

Edema localized in the eyelids may be the first sign of generalized edema.

Generalized Edema

Renal disease	Heart failure
Liver disease	Malnutrition
Systemic lupus erythromatosus	Adrenal hormones
Hyperaldosteronism	Thyroid disease
Infectious mononucleosis	

True, generalized pitting edema is found earliest over the dependent parts, especially the sacrum and ankles. Edema in the first few months of life may be seen in patients with cystic fibrosis. Adolescent girls show edema before or during menses. In warm weather, edema occasionally occurs on the skin without apparent cause.

Localized edema in the eyelids, face, or lips may be due to allergy (angioneurotic edema), sinusitis, trichiniasis (trichinosis), or insect bites in those areas. Puffiness of the eyelids may also be seen in children after a long sleep or after crying and in children with conjunctivitis, frontal or ethmoid sinusitis, cavernous sinus thrombosis, or infectious mononucleosis, or in those using illicit drugs. Edema of the face and eyelids is common in children with any of the common contagious diseases. Localized edema of the face may occur following severe cough, such as whooping cough or diphtheria. Facial edema also occurs with superior vena cava obstruction or mass lesions in the chest. Edema of the legs occurs with thrombophlebitis, deep calf vein thrombosis, inferior vena cava obstruction, cellulitis, and other lower extremity infections.

The ridges formed by the raised apertures of the sweat glands make up *dermatoglyphics*. These are best seen with adequate light and magnification or by making finger and hand prints. The otoscope without earpiece is usually adequate for both light and

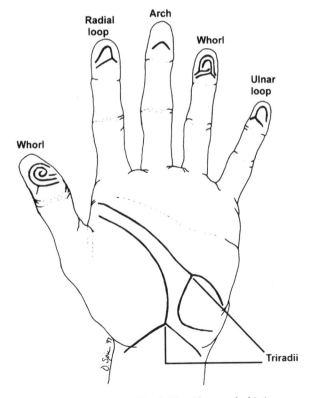

Figure 3-2. Normal hand ridges (dermatoglyphics).

magnification. The ridges form arches, loops, and whorls on the fingers; three lines that meet are termed triradii. The normal child usually has a triradius low on the palm, a triradius with an acute angle in the hypothenar area proximal to the midpalm, and an assortment of arches, loops, and whorls on the fingertips (Fig. 3-2). Usually, approximately seven or eight fingertips will have ulnar loops and one to three will have whorls. One arch is common in normal children. Radial loops are rare in normal children. Deviations from these patterns suggest the presence of chromosome abnormalities, early intrauterine infections, gross abnormalities of growth of the extremities, or some forms of congenital heart disease. A triradius distal to the midpalm with an obtuse angle is suggestive of Down syndrome; arches on all digits suggest trisomy 18 syndrome. Radial loops may occur more commonly in children with XXY anomaly, and large deep ridges are found in gonadal dysgenesis. Arches on the thumbs are common in children with trisomy 13 syndrome. A single flexion crease on the fifth finger suggests the presence of a chromosome abnormality.

NAILS

The *nails* are valuable areas for determining special disease states. The nail beds are usually the simplest site in which to determine cyanosis, pallor, capillary pulsations, and capillary refill time. In newborns, vernix can usually be found under the nails. Pitting of the nails is seen with fungal diseases of the nails and with psoriasis. Indentations (Beau's lines) are markers of previous severe stress. Yellow staining of the nails is apparent in postmature infants and in the yellow nail syndrome, which is associated with lymphedema and lung disease. Darkening of the nails may be noted in children with porphyria. Nails may be absent in children with ectodermal dysplasia or fetal alcohol syndrome or in infants born to mothers receiving anticonvulsants. Infections around the nails (paronychia) are common in children, especially after desquamating skin lesions. They may be bacterial or fungal infections. Oncolysis may indicate thyroid disease.

Hemorrhage under the nails is usually due to injury, subacute bacterial endocarditis, or other diseases in which petechiae are noted. Telangiectases at the proximal nail folds occur in scleroderma, lupus erythematosus, and dermatomyositis. Redness of the half-moon (lunula) occurs in children with heart failure, corticosteroid use, pulmonary disease, or alopecia areata. Brown discoloration of the lunula may occur in children with uremia.

The nail beds are characteristically more broad than long in children with Down syndrome or pseudohypoparathyroidism or in congenital malformation syndromes characterized by broad fingers. Spoon-shaped nails with loss of the longitudinal convexity (koilonychia) may be caused by fungal infections, iron deficiency, trauma, or thyroid or intestinal diseases, or they may be congenital. White nails or paired white lines parallel to the nail base (Muehrcke lines) are seen in hypoalbuminemic states, zinc and vitamin B_6 deficiencies, and other types of malnutrition. Transverse white lines (Mees' lines) in the nails may occur several months after acute Kawasaki disease or other severe illnesses.

Compare the width of thumbnails, first fingernails, and great toes. These may be the easiest sites in which to detect asymmetry or hemiatrophy.

HAIR

Note hair, other than that of the head. Newborns, especially premature infants, sometimes have hair growing over their shoulders and back but it disappears at about 3 months of age. Children do not usually have hair except for scalp, eyebrows, and eyelashes until near puberty. Long eyebrows and eyelashes are usually familial but occasionally appear in children with chronic or wasting diseases. Heavy facial hair occurs with de Lange and Hurler syndromes, which are associated with developmental delay, or in endocrine disorders such as virilizing tumors, polycystic ovary syndrome, arrhenoblastoma, and acromegaly. Look for nits or crab lice (a sexually transmitted disease) in these areas.

Unusual hairiness elsewhere on the body, especially over the arms and legs, may be a normal variant or familial characteristic but may be found in children with hypothyroidism, vitamin A poisoning, chronic infections, phenytoin or diazoxide use, or hepatic porphyria. Those who are starving or have extreme weight loss, as with anorexia-bulimia, have lanugo-type hairiness. Hairiness of the trunk is noted in children with Cushing syndrome.

Tufts of hair anywhere over the spine and especially over the sacrum may have special significance. Although resembling a nevus, the hair may mark the site of a spina bifida occulta or spina bifida. Nevi may also be hairy.

Pubic hair begins to appear at 8–12 years of age (adrenarche), followed by axillary hair about 6 months later and by facial hair at about 6 months later still in boys. Appearance of hair in these areas indicates normal adrenal and testicular function. Decrease of hair in these areas may be due to hypothyroidism, hypopituitarism, gonadal deficiency, or Addison disease. Early appearance or increase of hair in these areas may be normal, especially in obese children.

Increased Body Hair

Obese
Adrenal hyperplasia
Adrenal tumor
Acanthosis nigricans

Central nervous system lesions
Pineal hamartoma
Testicular tumors
Ovarian tumors
Hyperinsulism
Polyostotic fibrous dysplasia

Ingestion
Stilbestrol
Testosterone
Anabolic steroids

Pigmented, coarse, curly, or crinkled pubic hair indicates increased hormonal production and is believed to indicate onset of sperm formation in boys (Fig. 3-3). Pubic hair without testicular growth suggests hypogonadism.

LYMPH NODES

Lymph nodes are generally examined during examination of the part of the body in which they are located. Routinely palpate occipital, postauricular, anterior and posterior cervical (Fig. 3-4),

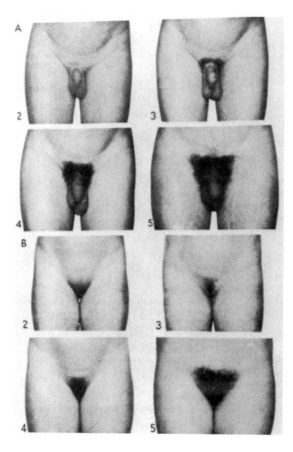

Figure 3-3. Pubic hair stages in males **(A)** and females **(B)**. Stage 1 (not shown): preadolescent (no pubic hair). Stage 2: sparse, long, slightly pigmented. Stage 3: darker, coarser, more curled. Stage 4: adult type but smaller area. Stage 5: adult. (From Tanner JM: *Growth at adolescence*. Philadelphia: F.A. Davis, 1962).

parotid, submaxillary, sublingual, axillary, epitrochlear, and inguinal nodes. Note size, mobility, tenderness, and heat. Shotty, discrete, movable, cool, nontender nodes up to 3 mm in diameter are usually normal in these areas; in the cervical and inguinal regions, nodes up to 1 cm in diameter are normal until age 12 years.

Nodes that are in the anterior cervical triangle or that enlarge slowly are usually benign. Rapidly growing nodes, nodes fixed to underlying tissue, or hard, firm, or matted nodes are usually malignant.

Large, warm, soft, tender nodes usually indicate acute infection. Firm, rubbery nontender nodes are more common with

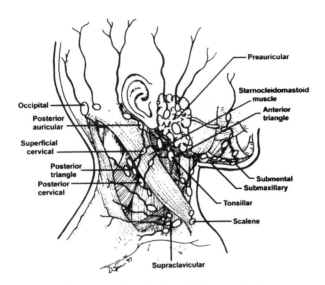

Figure 3-4.   Lymph nodes of the head and neck.

leukemia or sarcoid. Firm nodes that adhere to each other and the skin are found in children with tuberculosis; discrete rubbery nodes are found in Hodgkin disease, and extremely firm, hard nodes occur with metastases. Local adenopathy usually indicates local infection but may be a sign of generalized disease. Cervical nodes reflect drainage of the sinuses, ears, mouth, teeth, and pharynx. The right supraclavicular nodes drain the lung and esophagus; the left supraclavicular nodes drain the lung, stomach, small intestine, kidney, and pancreas; and the axillary nodes drain the breasts, arms, and fingers. In children with inguinal adenopathy, investigate for sexually transmitted diseases or paragenital infections.

Generalized adenopathy with or without tenderness is seen with systemic diseases.

Generalized Adenopathy

Bacteremia	Viremia
Syphilis	Kawasaki disease
Eczema	Leukemia
Infectious mononucleosis	Serum sickness
Systemic fungal disease	Hodgkin disease
Hyperthyroid	Sarcoid
Chronic granulomatous disease	Hyper-IgE
Drug sensitivity	Reticuloendothelial disease
Lupus erythematosus	
Rheumatoid arteritis	

A few isolated enlarged nodes may have special significance. Occipital or posterior auricular adenopathy is evident in local scalp infections, external otitis, German measles, pediculosis, varicella, tick bite, and in cases of excessive scratching. Posterior occipital nodes are frequently palpable in other viral infections but are rarely so in bacterial infections in the throat. The preauricular nodes may be enlarged in conjunctivitis (Parinaud syndrome) or in children with sties or chalazion. The "sentinel" node located near the left clavicle may be the first node enlarged in Hodgkin disease in children; in adults, this nodal enlargement may indicate gastric cancer. Cervical adenopathy usually accompanies acute infections in or around the mouth or throat, but cool, large, nontender, matted, cervical glands that may suppurate (especially if unilateral) may indicate tuberculosis. Cervical or submandibular lymph node enlargement without other symptoms may herald sinus histiocytosis. When adenopathy occurs near a scratch or bite, cat-scratch or rat-bite fever or tularemia is suggested, as is disease resulting from tick, flea, or mite bites or local sepsis. The epitrochlear nodes in particular are enlarged in congenital syphilis and cat-scratch disease.

Absence of lymph nodes occurs in patients with agammaglobulinemia and in some patients with human immunodeficiency syndromes.

Head and Neck

The head and neck grow rapidly in the first few years of life and alter the appearance of the child from infancy to childhood and throughout adolescence.

HEAD

By age 1 month, the infant in a prone position will usually hold the head dorsally. At 3 months of age, the normal infant holds the head steady when held upright by the physician. Failure to hold the head up usually indicates poor motor development. Head nodding may be normal, but it is usually seen in children who are emotionally unstable or mentally retarded or who have spasmus nutans.

Note amount, color, and texture of the *hair*. The newborn infant usually has hair that is fully replaced beginning at about 3 months of age. Lack of hair (alopecia) may be a familial characteristic or a manifestation of ectodermal dysplasia, hyperthyroidism, or progeria. Localized alopecia (alopecia areata) is seen in ringworm or other infections of the scalp and in acrodynia, but in infants it is most commonly caused by rubbing of localized areas when the infant lies in one position for a long time. Rarely, alopecia areata is seen in children with syphilis or hypervitaminosis A or in neurotic children who pull out the hair or occurs after severe systemic disease (e.g., typhoid fever). Other causes include the following:

Other Causes of Alopecia Areata

Exposures
- X-ray
- Caustics

Neoplasms
- Lymphoma
- Carcinoma
- Mycosis fungoides

Skin Diseases
- Bullous dermatoses
- Sarcoid
- Discoid lupus
- Leprosy
- Exfoliate dermatoses
- Acrodermatitis enteropathica

Other
- Collagen diseases (such as scleroderma)
- Scalp infections
- After antimetabolite or heparin therapy
- Arsenic or thallium poisoning
- Thyroid disease
- Iron biotin deficiency

Hair is normally smooth and of fine texture. Children with hypothyroidism, hypoparathyroidism, ringworm of the scalp, and arginosuccinicaciduria, a rare inborn error, have brittle hair. Fine hair may be seen in any of the states causing alopecia. Fine hair distinguishes hypopituitarism from primary thyroid disease, in which the hair is coarse and brittle. Hair that is either twisted, irregularly constricted, woolly, or irregularly pigmented may be inherited as an isolated anomaly. Children with the inborn metabolic condition of Menkes' kinky hair disease have steely hair. Examine the hair for the presence of pediculi or nits.

Note the *shape* of the head and face. Children with premature or irregular closure of the sutures exhibit marked *asymmetry* of the head. Flattening of part of the head or face occurs in an infant who lies in only one position or who has unusually soft bones. In children with rickets or delayed physical or mental development, the back of the head is flat. One side of the head and face is also flattened in children with torticollis or may appear flattened in children with facial palsy.

Examine the *scalp*. Special lesions may be noted in newborns. Scaling and crusting of the scalp, if generalized, are usually due to seborrheic dermatitis or eczema; if localized, they are caused by ringworm. Note infections of the scalp. Lymph nodes and subcutaneous nodules are identified by careful palpation, especially around the occiput.

Palpate the *sutures*. Usually, they are felt as ridges until infants are about 6 months of age. Note abnormal sutures, fractures, and fontanels. The posterior fontanel closes by the second month; the anterior fontanel usually closes by the end of the second year (Fig. 4-1).

Note the size and shape of the anterior fontanel by pressing lightly in the area of the opening. Normal infants aged less than 6 months of age occasionally may have a large fontanel (more than 4–5 cm in diameter), but it may also be diagnostic of chronically increased intracranial pressure, subdural hematoma, rickets, hypothyroidism, and osteogenesis imperfecta.

A tenseness or bulging of the fontanel is best noted if the patient is sitting. The normal fontanel may feel questionably tense in the infant who is supine. Tenseness may be noted in the crying child but only during expiration; this physiologic bulging disappears when the patient relaxes or inspires. Persistent or true bulging or tenseness of the fontanel in the quiet infant in the sitting position usually accompanies an acute increase in intracranial pressure.

Bulging Fontanel—Pseudotumor Cerebri

Meningitis
Brain tumor
Pulmonary insufficiency
Vitamin A excess
Cortisone withdrawal
Lateral sinus thrombosis
Cardiac failure

Lead poisoning
Retinoic acid
Tetracycline
Nalidixic acid
Subdural hematoma
Roseola

The fontanel is depressed in children with dehydration and malnutrition. A small fontanel is usually normal but is also an

Anterior

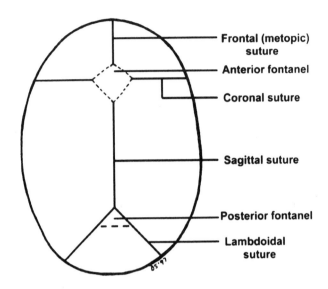

- Frontal (metopic) suture
- Anterior fontanel
- Coronal suture
- Sagittal suture
- Posterior fontanel
- Lambdoidal suture

Posterior

Figure 4-1.   Diagram of the top of the head indicating position of fontanels and palpable sutures.

important sign of microcephaly in infants. Occasionally, the fontanel is closed with only fibrous tissue and will feel less firm than the surrounding skull. Fibrous closure should be noted, but physiologically it is comparable to an open fontanel. Bony closure usually occurs 1–2 months after fibrous closure. Closure of the fontanel may be delayed in children with hydrocephalus, rickets, or cretinism. Rarely, delayed closure is due to syphilis or the osteochondrodystrophies.

Slight pulsations of the anterior fontanel occur in normal infants. However, marked pulsations may be a sign of increased intracranial pressure, venous sinus thrombosis, obstruction of the venous return from the head, or increased pulse pressure due to arteriovenous shunt, patent ductus arteriosus, or excitement. Aortic regurgitation is a rare cause of increased pulse pressure during the age when the fontanel is open.

Measure the circumference of the head. Until the child is 2 years of age, the circumference of the head is approximately the same as or slightly larger than that of the chest. Marked disproportions between the head and chest measurements indicate microcephaly, macrocephaly, or hydrocephaly. If the child's measurements are disproportionate, compare head and chest measurements with standards, since the chest itself may be large or small.

Microcephaly may be due to cerebral dysgenesis alone or to premature closure of the sutures (craniostenosis). Children with general growth failure rarely exhibit microcephaly.

Hydrocephalus, caused by chronic increase in intracranial pressure, is detected by noting an enlarged head, enlarged fontanel, supraorbital bulging, and open sutures. Dilated scalp veins are characteristic of early hydrocephalus. Hydrocephalus is an enlargement of the ventricular systems of the brain and may be due to blocking of the ventricular foramina (noncommunicating), blocking of the subarachnoid pathways (communicating) or, rarely, failure of the subarachnoid system to absorb cerebrospinal fluid (CSF: external).

Bulging of an area of the head occasionally occurs with brain tumors, lacunar defects of the skull, and intracranial masses. Bulging of the frontal areas (bossing) is characteristic of prematurity, rickets and, occasionally, congenital syphilis.

Craniotabes is best detected by pressing the scalp firmly just behind and above the ears in the temporoparietal or parietoooccipital region. Elicitation of a ping-pong ball-snapping sensation indicates craniotabes. It represents a softening of the outer table of the skull. Although infants with craniotabes sometimes cry, no danger is involved if the pressure is not so excessive that the inner table is pressed. Craniotabes is found in premature infants, in some normal children aged less than 6 months of age, in babies who lie constantly on one side of the head, and in children with rickets, syphilis, hypervitaminosis A, and hydrocephalus.

Macewen's sign is one that many physicians like to elicit, but it usually has little significance in childhood. On percussing the skull, you hear a resonant "cracked-pot" sound. As long as the fontanel is open, this type of sound is physiologic. After closure of the fontanel, the sound indicates increased intracranial pressure or a dilated ventricle.

Percuss the head in children with neurologic disorders in the indirect manner similar to that described for percussion of the heart. When the head is carefully percussed, you can occasionally elicit dullness near the sagittal sinus. This is a good sign of subdural hematoma.

Tenderness or pain over the occiput may indicate the presence of brain tumor or abscess. Pain over the scalp may accompany cerebral hemorrhage, migraine, trauma, hypertension, vascular neuralgia, anxiety, or depressive states. Press hard over the malar bones for a few seconds and then release. Functional headaches may be improved by this maneuver, but headaches with other causes will not change.

In children aged more than 2–3 years of age, percuss the frontal and maxillary *sinuses* in the same manner or by the direct method for tenderness. Tenderness indicates acute sinusitis. Swelling or tenderness elicited by pressure deep in the bony angle above the inner canthus of the eye is characteristic of acute ethmoiditis. It is difficult and generally unnecessary to transilluminate the sinuses in young children. The maxillary sinuses can be transilluminated after they are developed (see box).

Development of Sinuses		
Sinus	**Present**	**Developed**
Ethmoid	Birth	3 yr
Maxillary	Birth	3 yr
Sphenoid	3 yr	12 yr
Frontal	8 yr	12 yr
Mastoid	Birth	3 yr

Auscultation over the skull with the bell stethoscope may reveal a swishing sound (*bruit*) of blood flowing through dilated vascular channels. Systolic or continuous bruits may be heard normally in children until age 4 years or in children with anemia; after this age, systolic bruits suggest the presence of vascular anomalies, especially arteriovenous aneurysms, or increased intracranial pressure. Similar noise is sometimes heard in children with meningitis. Transmitted cardiac murmurs may sometimes be heard as bruits over the skull. Press over the carotid artery. The bruit disappears if it is *not* due to aneurysm.

Determine direction of blood flow in the scalp veins in children with suspected intracranial abnormalities. You may need to shave the scalp first to determine blood flow, but this procedure occasionally reveals abnormal vascularity or vascular channels indicative of underlying abnormalities. Small ossification defects through which the dura protrudes may occur in the skull. Small defects are termed *lückenschädel*, and large defects are termed *encephaloids*. Nerve tissue protrudes in children with encephaloceles. Encephaloceles may be present anywhere in the skull and are sometimes apparent near the inner canthus of the eye. On the shaved scalp, note also the presence of dimples, which may be an indication of a dermal sinus or hemangiomas. These are infrequent but sometimes remediable causes of seizures or meningitis. Scalp veins may appear dilated in very young infants; they also may indicate the presence of hydrocephalus, tumors, subdural hematoma, or congenital vascular anomaly.

Transilluminate the skull of children suspected of having intracranial lesions. Hold the otoscope light so that a tight fit is made with the child's scalp. The room must be quite dark. A sharply delineated area of increased light transmission may be noted over a subdural hygroma. Place a bright light at the occiput of infants suspected of having anencephaly. The light is transmitted through the eyes in anencephalic infants, and you will observe this response as pinkness of the retina.

FACE

Note the *shape* of the face. An easy way to determine *facial paralysis* is to observe the child while it is crying, whistling, or smiling. The paralyzed or weakened side will remain immobile, and the innervated side will wrinkle. The lips will rise only on the intact side, and the angle of the mouth may droop on the paralyzed side. Wrinkling of the forehead should be noted.

Unilateral paralysis of the face excluding the muscles of the forehead indicates a central facial nerve (supranuclear) weakness and may be seen in children with cerebral palsy or other brain lesions. Unilateral paralysis of the face including the muscles of the forehead and eyelid indicates a peripheral facial nerve lesion and may be due to trauma, otitis media, viral infections, Lyme disease, or other peripheral lesions. Recovery from peripheral facial nerve palsy may occur in the upper portion of the face first and, at this point, the palsy may resemble a supranuclear weakness. Bilateral facial diplegia is a characteristic of Guillian-Barré syndrome.

Salivary flow can be measured by placing polyethylene tubes in the submaxillary ducts. Stimulate salivation by placing a slice of lemon on the tongue. Count the drops that occur in 1 minute. If measured in a child with peripheral facial palsy, salivary flow will be at least 40% of normal in those palsies that spontaneously recover.

Paralysis and asymmetry about the mouth only are usually caused by a peripheral trigeminal nerve lesion with weakness of the masseter muscles. Jaw strength can be tested by asking the child to bite on a tongue depressor on each side of the mouth. Beware of the possibility of malocclusion, which may give the impression of weakness.

Trismus (contracture of the facial muscles) gives the child a sardonic smile (risus sardonicus), which occurs in tetany caused by hypocalcemia, tetanus, or phenothiazine sensitivity and may occur with streptococcal pharyngitis.

Local swellings about the face are usually due to edema. Edema only in the face may be due to any of the causes of generalized edema, as well as allergy (see Chapter 3). However, enlargement of the mandible in infants may be due to infantile cortical hyperostosis (Caffey syndrome) or vitamin A poisoning and may be mistaken for parotitis. Large jaws due to fibrous swelling with upward turning of the eyes is seen in cherubism. A small mandible (micrognathia) is usually a congenital anomaly but may be seen in children with rheumatoid arthritis.

To determine local swelling of the *parotid* glands, sit the child upright, ask the child to look toward the ceiling, and note the swelling below the angle of the jaw. Next, run the flat part of your finger downward from the zygomatic arch. The swollen parotid is then felt. Confirm it by telling the child to lie supine. The parotid falls back like jelly and pushes the pinna of the ear forward.

Parotid Swelling

Mumps	Allergy
Stone in parotid duct	Leukemia
Blowing balloon or wind instrument	Starch eaters
Bacterial infections in debilitated children	Persistent vomiting
	Sarcoid

Parotid swelling with lacrimal duct swelling is Mikulicz syndrome. Tumors and cysts occasionally occur in the parotid area in children. Firm swelling of the parotids (parotid sialadenitis) is usually self-limited; it may be caused by animal scratch diseases

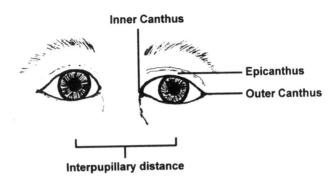

Figure 4-2. Measuring interpupillary distance.

or may be seen in children who compulsively eat starch. Nontender parotid swelling may precede the onset of diabetes mellitus. Enlargement of the masseter muscles may be mistaken for parotid swelling and occurs in bubble-gum addicts or binge eaters, such as bulimic patients.

Palpate the area under the jaw for *glands* or tenderness. Submaxillary glands are felt best by palpating lightly just below the mandible, anterior to the angle of the jaw, or by lightly rubbing this area with the fingertips. Sublingual glands are similarly palpated just behind the bony portion of the chin. These glands are ordinarily not palpable, and enlargement or tenderness usually indicates mumps, cystic fibrosis, local infection or infection in the teeth or, rarely, stones in the ducts. Recurrent swelling occurs with Sjögren syndrome. Unilateral submandibular or submaxillary swelling is more common with atypical mycobacteria, and bilateral swelling is more common with human tubercle bacilli.

Abnormal or unusual facial appearance is also seen in many children with generalized dystrophies, and some of these conditions have characteristic facies. Congenital abnormalities may be seen. Coarse facial features occur in children with mucopolysaccharidoses, hypothyroidism, multiple sulfatase deficiency, I cell disease, Job syndrome, other gangliosidoses, and Coffin-Siris syndrome.

Hypertelorism appears as a large distance between the eyes and occurs with a broadened nasal bridge. It is measured as an increased interpupillary distance and reflects the spacing of the orbits. It is due to overdevelopment of the lesser wing of the sphenoid bone. If the medial canthus is displaced laterally, *telecanthus*, a similar appearance may exist. Both conditions may be normal variants. Hypertelorism with other midfacial anomalies usually occurs in children who are mentally normal. If hypertelorism is extreme or occurs with anomalies other than those of the head and face, the probability of mental retardation is considerable.

Infants with *hypotelorism* and midface anomalies are almost always retarded. The normal interpupillary space is approximately 3.5–5.5 cm (Fig. 4-2). For small eyes, measure the palpebral fissure (the distance between the inner and outer canthus) with a tape. For premature infants, this fissure normally measures about 1.5 cm at 32 weeks of gestation and increases to about 1.8 cm for term infants. Infants with fetal alcohol syndrome have shortened palpebral fissures.

Twitchings of the face are usually due to tics or habit spasms, but they may be caused by muscular exhaustion or fasciculation.

To obtain Chvostek sign, tap the cheek of the child just below the zygoma with your finger. If the sign is present, that side of the face will grimace. It is difficult to elicit Chvostek sign in children under 2 weeks of age or in children who are crying. Chvostek sign may be present in normal children under 1 month or over 5 years of age. If this sign is present in children between these ages, it indicates hyperirritability and may be found with tetanus, tetany, and hyperventilation.

EYES

> *A baby's eyes—*
> *Their glance might cast out pain and sin,*
> *Their speech make dumb the wise*
> *By mute glad God-head felt within*
> *A baby's eyes.*
>
> *Source unknown*

The eye is not only the most important sensory organ, but is also a window to the brain. A careful examination of the eyes of a small child is basically made without the cooperation of the child and is difficult. Infants aged less than 1 year may be kept quiet with a bottle, but for children 1–4 years of age, you must use other wiles.

Even in a small child, the examination is best performed if you use your left hand carefully. Hold the ophthalmoscope in your right hand and keep your left hand far from the patient's eye to attract attention. The natural tendency is to try to hold the eye open forcibly. This results only in a wet eye that is impossible to hold open, a distraught child, and an overheated examiner. If the child starts to cry when the light approaches the eye, put the light away or let the child play with it and perform this part of the examination later.

The *sclera* is the white of the eye; the *cornea* is the pigmented area. The clear area of the cornea is round. A small pigmented curtain, (the iris) normally is also round and, by constricting and relaxing, it controls the amount of light that penetrates to the retina and through the pupil. The space inside the iris is designated the pupil (Fig. 4-3).

Vision may be assessed in very young children by noting the child's interest in a light or bright object and noting the pupillary response to light. A newborn sees only light; by 1 month of age, an infant can see smaller objects and by 2 months of age can see rough outlines and follow moving fingers. By 6 months of age, the infant should focus for short periods but is farsighted. In older children, vision can be estimated by the child's interest in brightly colored objects in the room. The eye may be examined by having the child fix, if even for a moment, on some familiar object such as the parent's nose or face. Apparent blindness in a child aged less than 4 months may be due to developmental delay.

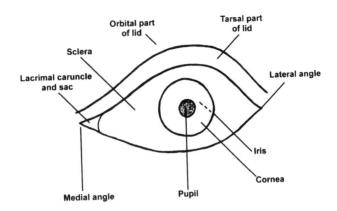

Figure 4-3.   The eye.

If more detailed tests of vision are desired in young children, they should be made before one proceeds further with the examination of the eye. Infants can respond to light and darkness. Observe children aged 1–2 years while they pick up different-sized colored objects from the floor. You can test a child older than 2 years with a letter E chart by asking the child which way the bars point. At age 3–5 years, both the child's eyes should see at least 20/40 and, after 5 years, 20/30 in both eyes, with no more than a two-line difference between eyes. The infant may also be tested by rotating a cylinder on which black and white lines are painted. An infant who sees will develop nystagmus as the cylinder is rotated; the blind infant's eyes will remain stationary. This cylinder test is also useful in distinguishing hysterical from organic blindness in older children. Blindness or varying degrees of decreased visual acuity may be due to optic nerve lesions, lesions anywhere in the eye including refractive errors, cortical atrophy, or CNS defects. Occasionally, temporary blindness may occur after head trauma, with no sequelae. Unilateral visual defect should direct your attention to lesions that are peripheral to the optic chiasm and in the eye.

If there is any question of a brain lesion, test *visual fields* by confrontation. Hold a piece of cotton in your hand, sit opposite the child, and have the child cover one eye while you close your eye. The child then looks at your open eye. Hold the cotton at arm's length and slowly bring it in, moving it through various planes midway between the child and you toward your eyes. As soon as the cotton is seen, the child will make a sudden movement toward it. This should occur at about the same time you see the cotton. Younger children may be asked to pick up small bright objects.

Vertical defects are termed *vertical hemianopia*. Heteronymous defects are almost always bitemporal, due to pressure on optic fibers at the chiasm. Homonymous defects usually indicate lesions posterior to the chiasm or in the visual cortex; temporal defects usually indicate lesions near the chiasm. Sudden onset of blind spots (scotoma) that enlarge and then resolve may be an

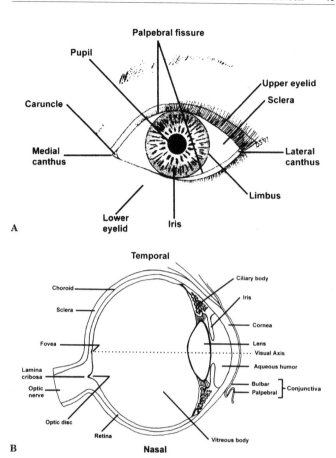

Figure 4-4. Normal structure of the eye. A: Frontal view of eye. B: Section through the orbit.

early sign of migraine. Central scotoma may be due to pressure on the chiasm or to poisons. Constricted visual fields that are fixed in size, regardless of the distance from the patient, may be caused by hysteria.

The next part of the routine eye examination consists of *observation* of the eye (Fig. 4-4). *Blinking* normally occurs bilaterally when a quick movement is made toward the eyes or when one cornea is touched. This is the basis of the corneal reflex. Spasmodic blinking is usually due to habit spasm.

The sclerae should be completely white, but they are blue in many normal children because of the normal thinness of the sclera. Children with osteogenesis imperfecta, iron deficiency, and Ehlers-Danlos syndrome have blue sclerae. Yellow or mud-colored sclerae may be the first sign of clinical jaundice. Red sclerae occur with conjunctivitis or may be due to drug or alcohol abuse. In carotenemia, the skin is yellow but the sclerae are clear. The top of the sclera is visible below the upper eyelid in children with the "setting sun" sign, which may be noted in normal premature infants, at times in normal full-term infants, and in some with abuse of phencyclidine. If marked, it is suggestive of hydrocephalus, increased intracranial pressure, or kernicterus. The bulbar conjunctiva covers the sclera.

Note *exophthalmos* or *enophthalmos*. Suspect exophthalmos if the eye appears large or protruding. Exophthalmos due to lid retraction occurs with hyperthyroidism, which is rare in childhood. In children with exophthalmos, the distance from the angle of the eye to the front of the cornea is more than 15 mm. Exophthalmos may be unilateral. The eyes may appear to bulge.

Apparent Bulging: Proptosis

Congenital glaucoma
Glaucoma
Orbital cellulitis, abscess
Retroorbital tumors, hemorrhage, metastases
Orbital tumors, optic glioma
Hand-Schüller-Christian disease
Neurofibromatosis
Lymphangioma, hemangioma
Cerebral sinus thrombosis
Hyperthyroidism

Suspect enophthalmos if the eye appears sunken or small. Enophthalmos is usually due to cervical sympathetic nerve damage, as in Horner syndrome or microphthalmos, but apparent retraction of the eyeballs is observed in children with chronic malnutrition or acute dehydration.

Note the position of the eyes at rest. When the child looks straight ahead, the irises should be between the lids. The iris may appear to be beneath the lower lid in children with the setting-sun sign.

Note *strabismus*. The eyes should be parallel when the child glances in any direction. If there is less parallelism when the eyes move in one direction, suspect muscle paralysis. If the deviation from parallelism is equal when the eyes move in all directions, the squint is nonparalytic or concomitant. An easy method of observing squint is to look at the eyes when the child is looking toward a light about 3 feet away. The reflection of the light should come from approximately the same part of each pupil.

Degree of strabismus can be estimated by degree of deviation of light reflection from the center of the pupil. Deviation is approximately 15 degrees if the reflection appears at the edge of the pupil, 30 degrees if the reflection is halfway between the edge of the pupil and the limbus (outer edge of the cornea), and 45 degrees if the reflection is at the edge of the limbus.

Another simple test for squint is the cover test. Hold a light about 2–3 feet from the child's eyes and sit directly in front of the child. Ask the child to focus on the light. Then cover one eye; the opposite eye is noted for motion. That eye is then covered, and the first eye is noted for motion. Motion indicates the presence of strabismus or tropia. Eye dominance can be determined by noting which eye moves a little during the cover test. Resistance to movement on covering of one eye more than the other may be an indication of defective central vision in one eye.

In strabismus, one eye (monocular) or both eyes (alternating) may be involved. Involvement can be determined by the constancy of the deviation in the cover test. Strabismus may be present only when the patient is tired (intermittent). Test for strabismus with distant and near objects. Squint may be present for only one of these planes of focus and still be concomitant.

In children with paralytic strabismus, the involved eye does not complete the full range of motion (ROM). In nonparalytic strabismus, each eye can move to all quadrants, but the eyes do not move simultaneously. Paralytic strabismus also occurs with retrobulbar pain and otitis in children with petrositis. Always check the child's vision carefully when strabismus is present, especially for equality of vision in both eyes.

Strabismus

Paralytic	Nonparalytic
Lesion of third, fourth, or sixth cranial nerve	Unilateral refractive error
	Nonfusion
Meningitis	Focusing difficulties
Botulism	Anatomic differences in eyes
Increased intracranial pressure	
Muscle weakness	

Strabismus is frequently present in newborns, but should be minimal after 6 months of age. Even in very young children, however, fixed strabismus needs a careful ophthalmologic examination to exclude lesions that cause limitation of vision, such as optic atrophy, tumor, and chorioretinitis. Large epicanthal folds partly cover the globe of the eye and may be confused with squint. A unilateral epicanthal fold may be associated with torticollis.

Loss of *upward gaze* may be a sign of generalized increased intracranial pressure, pineal tumor, or lesions in the superior colliculi (Parinaud syndrome). It may be a late sign of kernicterus. Slow movements of the eyes may be observed in any condition causing paresis or paralysis of the eye muscles or with hyperthyroidism. In comatose patients, deviation of the eye downward and laterally with the pupil dilated suggests cranial nerve dysfunction with tentorial herniation. In such patients, rotate the head quickly. Eyes normally show conjugate movements to the side opposite to the direction of rotation. Absence of this response (doll's eye sign) indicates brainstem or oculomotor nerve dysfunction.

Note *nystagmus* by observing the constant motion of the eyes. Rarely, attempt to induce horizontal nystagmus by having the patient focus on an object from the outer angle of the eye. Record the direction of the fast and slow components of the nystagmus, as well as whether the nystagmus is spontaneous or induced. Circular, elliptical, and latent nystagmus are congenital. Rotatory nystagmus suggests a lesion in the medulla.

In infancy, spontaneous nystagmus may occur in hypothyroidism or may be congenital or of unknown etiology. The infant may be blind and have a peculiar searching type of nystagmus. Nystagmus is characteristic of cerebellar lesions and brain tumors and also occurs in the degenerative neurologic diseases and vestibular diseases. Vestibular nystagmus is always jerky, not pendular. The fast jerks are directed away from the involved ear. It may be evident in children with severe refractive errors. Bilateral, asymmetric nystagmus, pronounced in one eye and hardly discernible in the other, may be a sign of spasmus nutans. It is found in those who consume such drugs as marijuana, alcohol, benzodiazepines, or phencyclidine. Nystagmus present in a child with the eyes shut is congenital or should be considered vestibular in origin. Seesaw nystagmus, in which one eye moves rhythmically up while the other goes down, suggests a lesion near the third ventricle.

Ptosis of the lid may be congenital. It may represent birth injury to the brain or peripheral oculomotor nerve. If it is associated with a sunken eyeball, constricted pupil, anhidrosis, and facial pallor, it is due to cervical sympathetic paralysis (Horner syndrome). Ptosis may be an early sign of myasthenia gravis, botulism, amyotonia congenita, and myotonic dystrophy and occurs in children with heroin use, encephalitis, or tendon injury to the levator palpebra superior. It may occasionally be noted in children recovering from tetany.

Only slight ptosis results from sympathetic paralysis. Third-nerve paralysis results in severe ptosis. Ptosis associated with automatic elevation of the lid during chewing (the jaw-winking or Gunn phenomenon) is a congenital anomaly. Because of weakness of the orbicularis oculi, the palpebral fissures are more widely spaced on the involved side in children with facial palsy.

Other abnormalities of the *eyelids* should be noted. Hemorrhagic discoloration of the lids may be due to injury, neuroblastoma, or any bleeding dyscrasia such as scurvy and leukemia. Distortion of the lid may be due to edema, retrobulbar tumor, or metastases such as neuroblastoma. Extensive infection of the lids may be due to deep abscess formation or osteomyelitis around the sinuses. Fistulas near the lids may be congenital or may be due to chronic infection. Hemangiomas of the lids are common. Violaceous eyelids may be noted in children with dermatomyositis and scleroderma. Crepitation of the lids (emphysema) is due to air trapping and may follow fracture of the nose or sinuses. Look for distichiasis, a congenital anomaly of the eyelids with double rows of eyelashes or occasional aberrant hairs.

Dark circles under the eyes may be noted. Their significance is uncertain, but they may indicate tiredness, insufficient sleep, or allergy, or they may be a residual of edema in the face. Infraorbital eyelid creases (Morgan's lines) are found in allergic children.

Examine the *conjunctivae* for inflammation, conjunctivitis, hemorrhages, and foreign body. Conjunctivitis alone does not usually produce severe pain—only burning, soreness, or itching. If a foreign body is suspected, use a magnifying lens with good lighting. Photophobia may be present with conjunctivitis. The usual causes of redness of the conjunctivae in childhood are:

Conjunctival Redness

Bacterial or viral infection ("pink eye")
Allergy
Foreign body
Crying
Marijuana smoke
Vitamin D poisoning
Measles
Kawasaki disease (bulbar)
Eye strain
Acrodynia
Erythema multiforme

An early sign of measles, seen occasionally even before Koplik spots appear in the mouth, is the appearance of small red transverse lines in the conjunctivae (Stimson lines).

Conjunctivitis is common in newborns and may be due to gonorrhea, chemical irritation, or inclusion blennorrhea, which is probably caused by *Chlamydia oculogenitale*. Noting the extent of the conjunctivitis is important. In gonorrheal conjunctivitis or with any acute iritis, the bulbar and palpebral conjunctivae are inflamed; in conjunctivitis due to chemical irritation, the bulbar conjunctivae are usually spared and only the palpebral conjunctiva are inflamed. Children with vitamin A deficiency manifest dry wrinkled conjunctivae with foamy, yellow patches (Bitot spots). Small comma-shaped vessels in the lower bulbar conjunctivae are characteristic of vascular stasis and sickle cell disease.

Small *hemorrhages* in the conjunctivae may be significant signs of bacterial endocarditis, scurvy, and meningococcemia. They are also seen in the bleeding diseases. They are commonly seen in the normal newborn and in children following cough or trauma.

Pingueculae are small, yellowish, wedge-shaped areas near the cornea. They occasionally occur with the xanthomatoses or Gaucher disease. *Pterygium*, a wing-shaped white area that may cover the cornea, is an abnormal extension of the conjunctiva.

Sties (hordeolum) usually occur on the lower lid as tender, reddish-yellow pustules at the root of the hair follicle. Recurrent sties may be a sign of eyestrain, exposure to dust or dirt, general debility, or hay fever, although a sty may be an early sign of diabetes. A nonpainful, yellow swelling of the eyelid edge (chalazion) is due to inclusion cyst. Scaling of the lid margins (blepharitis) may be due to seborrhea, allergy, or infection.

The *cornea* should be crystal clear and is best examined with good room illumination or with an open bulb placed about 2 feet in front of the patient. The cornea is about 10 mm in diameter at birth and about 12 mm at adulthood. Any inflammation, ulceration, or opacity is abnormal. The cornea is clear in a child with conjunctivitis.

Note redness of the cornea due to vessel engorgement. If the redness is less near the cornea and increases toward the conjunctiva, superficial inflammation (keratitis) is probably present. If redness is greater near the cornea and fades toward the periphery, deep (ciliary) inflammation (iritis) is present, and the eye is painful.

Opacities in the cornea are usually due to ulcerations. White, Swiss-cheeselike superficial membranes at the periphery of the cornea is band keratopathy due to deposition of calcium and is observed in children with hypercalcemia, chronic uveitis, or juvenile rheumatoid arthritis.

Yellow opacities usually indicate active ulcerations; bluish-white opacities are healed ulcerations. Note depth of ulceration. Active ulcerations are usually associated with pain, photophobia, redness of the eye, and a small pupil. If inflammation or opacity is present, suspect foreign body, trauma, or infection. Corneal ulceration may occur with riboflavin deficiency or may be due to herpes.

Pinhead grayish ulcerations with conjunctivitis (phlyctenular conjunctivitis) is a rare painful form of tuberculosis or tuberculin sensitivity. It begins at the corneal–scleral junction and then invades the cornea. Deep ciliary inflammation is especially common in children with interstitial keratitis due to late congenital syphilis. The entire cornea may appear steamy white. Keratoconjunctivitis also occurs with measles and other viral diseases and with rheumatoid arthritis. A gray-green-orange ring around the cornea—the Kayser-Fleischer ring—is seen in hepatolenticular degeneration (Wilson disease).

The cornea is hazy in children with glaucoma, drug abuse, or avitaminosis A, and in children with metabolic diseases such as mucopolysaccharidoses and cystinosis, although slitlamp examination is usually necessary to demonstrate crystal formation in the cornea. A large cornea may also be a sign of glaucoma.

Foreign bodies on the cornea or conjunctiva may be detected easily unless they lie over the pupil. If you suspect a foreign body, evert the lids and swing the light in different directions while carefully examining the eye. You will observe either the foreign body or its shadow. The eyelids can be everted by asking the patient to look down. Place an applicator stick just over the edge of the upper eyelid and pull the eyelid forward and upward. If the suspected foreign body or abrasion cannot be located, fluorescein sticks may be placed in the eye. On oblique illumination, the injured area of the cornea will stand out with a greenish fluorescence.

With the light in the same position, evaluate the anterior chamber. Blood or small white spots may be observed. Blood is usually due to injury. White spots may be an early sign of uveitis. Light sensitivity suggests iritis or keratitis.

Note *discharges* from the eye. An infant ordinarily does not have tears before 1 month of age, and the lacrimal duct opens several weeks later. A watery discharge in infancy, usually from one eye, may signify a blocked tear duct. Press on the tear sac, which is just below the inner canthus of the eye. At the same time, slightly evert the lower lid so that you can observe the small opening (punctum). If fluid escapes when you apply pressure, there may be obstruction below the lacrimal sac. Fixed, red, painful swelling and induration in the area of the lacrimal sac indicate abscess formation with blockage (dacryocystitis). Obstruction without infection is usually a congenital anomaly; with infections, it is an acquired disease. A bluish swelling over the lacrimal sac may be a dacryocystocele and should be differentiated from a hemangioma. Tearing with a wet nose, however, may be a sign of infantile glaucoma; when a tear duct is blocked the nose is usually dry.

Watery discharges (epiphora) are also seen with allergy, sinusitis, sties, and drug abuse. Purulent discharges are due to infections. In newborns, the pus due to the chemical irritants placed in the eye may easily be confused with gonorrheal ophthalmia. Absence of tears has been noted as a characteristic of children with familial dysautonomia or Sjögren syndrome.

The *iris* contains two muscles that control the size of the pupils and is usually blue at birth and becomes pigmented within 6 months. Inequality of pigmentation may be a congenital anomaly or may be due to metallic foreign bodies. In Horner syndrome, the involved side remains blue and the opposite side acquires pigment. Different-colored irises (heterochromia) may indicate Waardenburg syndrome. Observe the iris to determine any fluttering, which may occur with subluxation or detachment of the lens. Absence of a part of the iris (coloboma) may be associated with other anomalies or with Wilms' tumor. Adhesions may be seen from the iris toward the lens. These may be congenital, due to persistence of the pupillary membranes, or may occur with chronic iritis, as in rheumatoid arthritis. Black and white spots (Brushfield spots) in the iris are usually evident in children with Down syndrome. Pigmented nodules (Lisch nodules) are characteristic of children with neurofibromatosis. In the iris, nodules may be due to tuberculosis, and hypopigmented spots are evident in tuberous sclerosis. When a light shines on the iris of patients with albinism, the eye lights up as if a switch had been thrown.

Compare the *pupils* for size and shape. They should be round, regular, clear, and equal. The pupil controls the quantity of light reaching the retina, minimizes aberrations of the peripheral cornea and lens, and increases depth of field. Irregularities in the pupil are usually due to congenital malformations. The sudden appearance of an irregular pupil should make you immediately suspect a penetrating foreign body through the cornea. White bands over the pupil may be due to congenitally persistent pupillary membranes. Unequal pupils (anisocoria) are usually congenital, but if they appear suddenly in the presence of equal illumination, they usually indicate acute intracranial disease.

Note *reaction to light* of the pupils. Size and light reaction are controlled by the sympathetic nervous system and the parasympathetics carried by the third cranial nerve. Children's pupils should react to light quickly. Reaction of the pupil in which the light shines is the direct reaction. The reaction of the opposite pupil is the consensual reaction. Absence of consensual reaction on one side occurs with optic nerve or retinal lesion and on both sides with a midbrain lesion. The pupils of newborn infants are constricted until about 3 weeks of age, so light reaction, while always sluggish in an infant with congenital glaucoma, is not a good test of glaucoma in newborns. Acute pain or excitement may cause dilation of pupils.

A fixed, dilated pupil indicates sympathetic stimulation, blindness, or poisoning. It may be caused by pressure on the midbrain due to acute increase in intracranial pressure. It may indicate a homolateral extradural or subdural hematoma, or meningitis. Injury to the ciliary ganglion can result in a dilated pupil that reacts poorly to light but constricts to near accommodation (Adie pupil). This does not indicate intracranial injury and usually follows injury to the eye. Dilated, unreactive pupils are seen with atropine or deep barbiturate poisoning, cocaine or amphetamine use, or anoxia. Dilatation of the contralateral pupil on light stimulation of one eye suggests injury to the eye and poor vision of the opposite eye, even in a comatose or uncooperative patient (Marcus Gunn sign). Pupils that react to accommodation but not to light (Argyll Robertson pupils) indicate a midbrain lesion, as occurs in Lyme disease, viral encephalopathies, syphilis, and granulomatous diseases.

Dilated pupils do not react in children whose coma is due to compressing lesions of the brain, but they are usually reactive in comatose children with metabolic disease. The pupils remain dilated in children with partial blindness, but the pupils respond to light in children with cortical blindness. Pupils may react slowly or not at all in those consuming illicit drugs. The pupils do not react during a petit-mal episode, in contrast to those in children who are staring or daydreaming.

Constricted, unreactive pupils are noted in children with cervical sympathetic palsy (Horner syndrome) or acute iritis, or in opiate, light barbiturate, or cholinesterase enzyme poisoning. In neurosyphilis of childhood, the pupils remain fixed and small because of parasympathetic injury. Constricted pupils generally indicate that the third-nerve impulses are intact.

Hippus is exaggerated rhythmic contraction and dilatation of the pupils. It may be a normal variant but also occurs with CNS disease.

Accommodation can be tested even in young children by having them look first at a shiny colored object at a distance and quickly bringing the object toward the eye. The pupil contracts as the object is brought near the eye. This reaction is known as the *convergence reaction*. Various neurologic disorders, including diphtheria and alcohol and other drugs, cause loss of the accommodation reflex. Most infants are hyperopic, but occasionally very young infants will play with objects within 2–3 inches of their eyes. Such infants will probably be myopic when their vision develops fully.

Examine the *lens* with direct light from the unshaded bulb. White or gray spots usually indicate opacities (cataracts) in the lens. In persons with cataracts, almost nothing can be seen beyond the white membrane of the lens when a light shines into the eye (see box and Fig. 4-4B).

Successful *internal examination* of the eye depends on your having gained the confidence of the child and having learned to develop a picture image of what you see in a flash. (This same technique is useful in examination of the pharynx in children.) Tell the patient that the room will be darkened, that a light will shine in the eyes, but that nothing painful will be done. Eye drops should be avoided but may be necessary. If the child is old enough, ask the child to look at a brightly colored picture across the room. Children who are somewhat younger can be given a flashlight and asked to turn it on and shine it on the picture across the room.

First, use a +8 to +2 lens to examine the cornea, iris, and lens and then a 0 to –2 lens for examination of the disc and retina.

Causes of Cataracts in Infants and Children

Metabolic Disorders
  Galactosemia
  Galactokinase deficiency
  Diabetes mellitus
  Mannosidosis
  Hypoparathyroidism
  Homocystinuria
  Fabry disease
  Refsum disease
  Cerebrotendinous
    xanthomatosis
  Wilson disease
  Glucose 6-phosphatase
    deficiency

Renal Disorders
  Lowe syndrome
  Alport syndrome

Musculoskeletal Disorders
  Chrondrodysplasia
    punctata
  Myotonic dystrophy
  Stickler syndrome
  Robert syndrome

Congenital
  Retinopathy of
    prematurity
  Maternal diabetes
  Maternal thyroid disease
  Maternal parathyroid
    disease

Skin Disorders
  Cockayne syndrome
  Incontinentia pigmenti
  Ichthyosis

Craniofacial Disorders
  Hallermann-Streiff
    syndrome
  Smith-Lemli-Opitz
    syndrome
  Rubinstein-Taybi
    syndrome
  Marshall syndrome
  Cerebro-oculo-facial
    syndromes
  Chromosome
    abnormalities,
    including trisomy 21

Central Nervous System
  Marinesco-Sjögren
    syndrome
  Rubella syndrome

Ocular Disorders
  Retinoblastoma
  Glaucoma
  Trauma

Use your right eye to examine the patient's right eye and your left eye for the patient's left eye. Start about a foot away from the patient's eye and, as you approach the eye, change the ophthalmoscope lenses so that they become less positive. The retina is usually best visible with a 0 to –2 lens in infants and children and is usually seen first as a red area (the red reflex) (Fig. 4-5). The details become obvious as you move closer. With this type of illumination, opacities in the cornea, anterior chamber, or lens will usually be seen as black spots against the red reflex of the retina. The anterior chamber is hazy with iritis, shallow with glaucoma, and dark with blood (hyphema).

With direct light, pearly gray, opaque, round areas in the center of the lens are typical of cataracts. Lenticular cataracts are usually lamellar (zonular) in children.

The lens may appear clear but misshapen. The posterior eye structures will be seen with difficulty. The lens may be dislocated upward, as in patients with Marfan syndrome, or downward, as

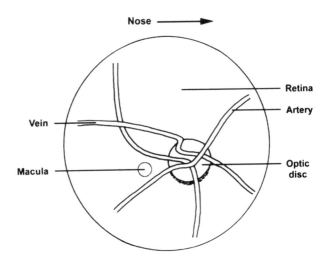

Figure 4-5.   Diagram of the retina.

in patients with homocystinuria. Other syndromes with dislocated lenses include Sturge-Weber, Ehlers-Danlos, Crouzon, Weill-Marchesani, sulfite oxidase deficiency, and mandibulofacial dysostasis.

The appearance of the *red reflex* from the retina provides important information. Ordinarily, the fundus will be pink and shiny, but it may be gray in deeply pigmented or in anemic children. The retina becomes gray and loses its shine whenever it becomes avascular. Absence of the red reflex or the appearance of a white-opaque reflex (leukokoria) is noted in children with opacities of the cornea or lens, cataracts, persistent posterior fibrovascular sheath of the lens, retrolental fibroplasia, retinal detachment, or retinoblastoma. Darkly pigmented freckles in the retina occur in children with familial polyposis; a lighter pigment may indicate retinitis pigmentosa, which is accompanied by the complaint of night blindness.

Veins and *arteries* are of almost equal size, or the veins are slightly larger than the arteries. In the hypertensive diseases, especially nephritis, the arteries are narrow. The vessels are dilated and cyanotic in children with cyanotic heart disease. Venous distention is an early sign of increased intracranial pressure. The veins pulsate normally. Exaggerated pulsations of the arteries, however, may indicate arteriovenous fistula, aortic regurgitation, or other causes of increased pulse pressure. All vessels of the disc are engorged with inflammation of the optic nerve (optic neuritis) and may appear small and thickened with arteritis, as in the collagen diseases.

Fresh *hemorrhages* on the retina in newborns may indicate trauma or anoxia or may be a cardinal sign of subdural hematoma. In older infants and children, fresh hemorrhages almost always indicate child abuse (shaken baby syndrome) but they are also seen in those with rare metabolic diseases, e.g., glutaric acidemia. They appear as red spots alone or with a surrounding white haze. These spots are also seen with sinus thrombosis, leukemia, scurvy, bacterial endocarditis, and other bleeding diseases. Multiple, gray, mulberrylike *tubercles* in the retina are seen in children with tuberous sclerosis, tuberculosis, and neurofibromatosis.

Patchy areas of white and red indicate *chorioretinitis*. They may appear in various infections but are characteristic of infection with toxoplasmosis, cytomegalic inclusion disease, syphilis, tuberculosis, and chronic brucellosis. Grayish-brown streaks radiating out from the disc are angioid streaks, seen in pseudoxanthoma elasticum.

The *disc* is most easily found if you relax and gaze from the temporal side of the patient's eye toward the posterior aspects of the eye. The edges of the disc usually have a sharp border around half the circumference and then fade. Blurring indicates increased intracranial pressure. The entire disc may be surrounded by a melanin ring, and this is usually normal. Gray stippling around the optic disc is a sign of lead poisoning. The disc is usually in the same plane as the retina in children. It is usually a little less pink than the surrounding retina. It is very pale in patients with anemia.

The disc may appear large and swollen, the edges may appear blurred, and the retinal vessels may appear to bend down from the disc to the retina in children with papilledema. Use the green filter to detect minimal blurring. Such "choked" or bulging discs indicate increased intracranial pressure or optic neuritis. Brain tumors or abscesses, except those originating in the anterior fossa, usually cause papilledema. Pulmonary insufficiency, especially that associated with obesity, may be associated with papilledema (a form of pseudotumor cerebri) (see list on p. 37).

The disc appears white in children with optic neuritis or optic atrophy.

White Optic Disc

Optic neuritis	Cystic fibrosis
Optic nerve atrophy	Thiamine deficiency
Meningitis	Brain tumors
Encephalitis	Optic nerve tumors
Generalized infections	Fibrous dysplasia
Neurofibroma	Poisons
Osteopetrosis	Septooptic dysplasia

It may precede other signs of multiple sclerosis, or it may be an isolated finding. Unilateral papilledema with contralateral optic atrophy may be due to a frontal lobe tumor (Foster-Kennedy syndrome). If the retina appears opalescent, retinal detachment may be present. Cupping of the disc in which the vessels appear to dip down from the retina toward the disc may be physiologic or may be exaggerated with glaucoma or in children with any of the conditions causing white disc.

Just to the temporal side of the disc is a small yellow-red area devoid of vessels—the *macula*. Because the macula is the most light-sensitive area of the eye, the pupil constricts as the macula is approached. In an older child, the macula can be visualized if

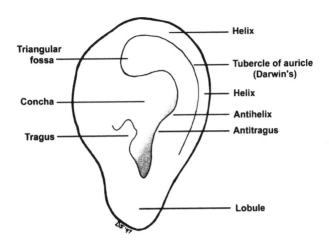

Figure 4-6.   The external ear.

the child is told to look at the ophthalmoscope light. This area appears to be cherry-red in reticuloendothelial diseases such as Tay-Sachs and Niemann-Pick disease and in other lysosomal storage diseases. The macula may be brown and appear fragmented in children with the juvenile form of macular degeneration. Bruit over the eyeball may occur with congenital arteriovenous fistulas in the brain.

Later in the examination, obtain the *corneal reflex* by touching the cornea with a piece of cotton or suddenly bring an object toward the child's eyes. Both eyes normally shut. Failure to obtain the corneal reflex indicates trigeminal (sensory component) or facial (motor component) nerve injury. Pontine injuries and anesthesia and many drugs depress this reflex.

In general, complete cooperation is impossible with young children. As the child grows older, devices for obtaining attention should be used. However, with or without the child's cooperation, you should explore these areas of the eye. If you note a defect in any area, refer the patient to an ophthalmologist, who can use other instruments and anesthetics.

EARS

Except in thermolabile children, the most common cause of fever without obvious reason in childhood is ear infection. Examine the ears of all sick children.

Various *anomalies* of the ears occur (Fig. 4-6). Obvious deformities of the auricle may be associated with other anomalies. Occasionally, a small sinus is present as a hole or pit just in front of the ear and this may be accompanied by a small swelling just inside the canal; this represents the remnant of the first brachial cleft. Large protruding auricles are a feature of children with fragile X syndrome. Lack of cartilage in the auricle may be a sign of relapsing polychondritis.

Note the *position* of the ears. In infants with Potter's syndrome, the tops of the ears are below the level of the eye and

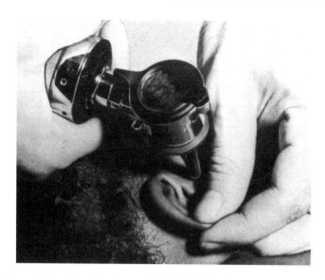

Figure 4-7. Using the otoscope. The hand holding the otoscope rests firmly on the patient's head or face.

there is congenital absence of the kidneys. Other gross anomalies of the ears may be associated with lesser kidney anomalies and with chromosome abnormalities.

The auricles frequently appear to stand forward with any mass or swelling behind the ear. Important conditions causing this appearance are mastoiditis, cellulitis, mumps, and postauricular abscesses. Occasionally, enlarged postauricular nodes or external otitis with surrounding cellulitis makes the ears protrude.

Note the nature and odor of discharge from the aural canals. A greenish, foul-smelling discharge occurs with pyocyanic infections. Purulent discharges are seen with any bacterial infection, particularly *Streptococcus pneumoniae* and *Mycobacterium tuberculosis*, but may also occur with fungal infections of the canal wall. Generalized eczema may cause flaking in the ears. Bloody discharge is usually due to scratching, irritation, or injury of the ear canal, but may occur with foreign body in the canal or be a cardinal sign of basilar skull fracture.

Next, use the otoscope (Fig. 4-7). First, use an otoscope that is halogen-illuminated and operating properly with fresh batteries or the light will turn yellow. Second, use the largest possible speculum. The speculum should never enter the canal more than 10–15 mm. Using the 1- or 2-mm speculum, even in infants, will only cloud the field and hurt the patient. Third, examine the canal before you try to look at the drum to note the presence of a furuncle or vesicle in the outer edge of the canal. If you hit a furuncle with the otoscope, the child will feel pain and the examination will probably end! Fourth, hold the otoscope firmly with one hand and, as the speculum is inserted, rest the hand holding the otoscope firmly on the child's head or face so that any motion by the child will be accompanied by a similar movement of the otoscope. Fifth, placing the speculum just inside the canal of one ear and then the other before attempting to examine the drum is also valuable. This assures the child that the procedure will not hurt. Examining the child's doll or the parent's ear first or pretending to look for an elephant in the child's ear may also reassure the child. Finally, before using the otoscope, remember the direction of the canal. In infants, the canal is directed upward, so the auricle should be pulled down to view the drum. In older children, the canal faces downward and forward; therefore, pull the tip of the auricle up and back for adequate visualization. Pulling the external ear serves another useful purpose. Ordinarily, this movement is painless in children with otitis media and in children without an ear infection, but it is painful in children with a furuncle in the ear or external otitis.

Examination of the ears should be almost painless. Allow the child to play with the otoscope, but handle the child firmly at the time of the examination. Either the child assures you of cooperation or the mother holds the child so that the head does not move and the hands do not interfere. The child should be placed face down and prone with the head turned first to one side, then the other. Tell the child that the speculum plays a song but that the child must be very quiet to hear it. After examining the first ear, ask the child if the song was heard. Then repeat the procedure in the opposite ear.

The *canal* and auricle may be swollen in children with external otitis, as occurs with seborrhea and allergic dermatitis or in nervous children who frequently place foreign bodies in the canal. Note any tenderness. Tenderness as the speculum is placed in the canal may indicate disease of the canal, such as a furuncle, or disease of the middle ear (otitis media). Vesicles in the canal may be due to viral canal infections or otitis media caused by *Haemophilus influenzae*. If cerumen is present, a large-enough speculum frequently allows you to look above or below the wax at the drum. If a small, easily reached foreign body or obstructive wax is present, it is best removed with an ear spoon or wire loop. You may see ear tubes in the drum or lying free in the canal.

Discharges may arise from the canal, external otitis, otitis media with perforation of the drum, or chronic otitis media with mastoiditis. Swimmer's discharge is usually due to Gram-negative bacilli. Greenish discharge is usually from external otitis. Mucoid or mucopurulent discharge most often arises from the middle ear. Carefully wipe away discharges with a soft, cotton-tipped applicator. Be careful to blot the discharge so that nothing is pushed against the ear drum, which may be perforated. Do not use cotton-tipped applicators to remove hard wax or foreign bodies.

Rarely, you may resort to use of an ear syringe to remove adherent wax. First, soften the wax with a detergent. Fit the syringe with a narrow "fistula tip" to provide a thin stream. Fill the syringe with lukewarm water (cover the patient to prevent soaking), and introduce it gently into the tip of the canal, which is then flushed. In examination of children, this procedure is unpleasant and undesirable because a vestibular response, frequently with vomiting, is induced. It should never be performed if perforation of the drum is suspected or if a foreign body is in the canal.

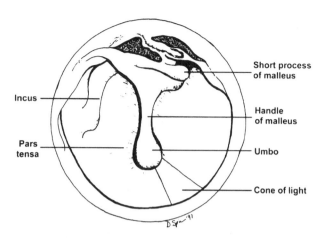

Figure 4-8. Diagram of the tympanic membrane.

The normal *drum* (Fig. 4-8) is gray-white and translucent or opalescent. The handle of the malleus appears as a small white streak running down and back to the center of the ear and ends at the umbo. At the upper end of the malleus is a small white projection, the short process of the malleus. Below the umbo is a small circle of light, the light reflex. Even in infants, in whom the drum is almost horizontal, determine these landmarks. As the child grows older, the drum becomes vertical but points inward. The light reflex becomes cone-shaped and sharply outlined, with the apex at the center and the base at the antero–inferior portion of the drum.

The most common abnormality of the drum noted on otoscopic examination is slight redness. This may be due to crying or to manipulation. If the drum is slightly to markedly reddened and retracted, as noted by the prominence of the malleus and a deeper and sharper outline of the cone of light, and if the vessels are prominent, "catarrhal" otitis media is present. This is usually due to any upper respiratory infection, usually viral, or to obstruction of the eustachian tube. The light reflex may appear less prominent than usual.

In acute suppurative otitis media, the *light reflex* is usually lost, the drum bulges outward and becomes diffusely red, the handle of the malleus is not clearly apparent, and hearing is usually decreased. Occasionally with a bulging drum, the light reflex is scattered diffusely over the drum area instead of being lost. Recognize that this reflex is coming from a convex drum, since the handle of the malleus is not observed. Otitis media in young infants may be due to congenital syphilis in addition to the usual causes of suppuration, such as *H. influenzae*, pneumococci, streptococci, staphylococci, and viruses. Otitis, sometimes with mastoiditis and abducens paralysis of the homolateral eye, occurs with petrositis (Gradenigo's syndrome). Chronic otitis may be due to tuberculosis or other bacterial infections, immune defects, allergy, and histiocytosis. It may also be associated with enlarged adenoids, cleft palate, and mastoiditis. Infants who have been fed frequently with a propped bottle or in the supine position may have otitis.

Bulging may also be due to nonpurulent fluid. This occurs in children with late catarrhal otitis media or suppurative otitis in which the bacterial infection has resolved but the exudate has not yet been resorbed (serous otitis). Bulging with a bluish discoloration of the drum may be due to a collection of blood in the middle ear and occurs after trauma and sometimes after infections. Blood behind the drum suggests basilar skull fracture.

The drum may be *perforated*. Perforation with pus indicates acute or chronic purulent otitis media. Small perforations may be seen in the drum due to injury, insect bites, or chronic tuberculosis. You may prefer to quantitate the conducting mechanism of the ear by tympanometry, which helps document fluid in the inner ear, drum perforation, and other changes in air and sound conduction.

Myringitis may be indicated if you find varying degrees of redness of the drum, with possibly some loss of the light reflex but without bulging or retraction or evidence of fluid in the middle ear, especially if associated with exquisite pain and little hearing loss. Myringitis is a primary inflammation of the drum head without involvement of the middle ear or may be an early stage of otitis media.

Occasionally, you will see a small spherical mass (usually gray, red, or yellow) just in front of or behind the drum: a cholesteatoma (Fig. 4-9). A pinpoint perforation may accompany it in the posterosuperior or central portion of the drum.

Note *mobility* of the drum. This requires a tight-fitting otoscope and speculum with a hole through which a puff of air can be introduced with an attached rubber bulb. Another option is to attach a tube to the otoscope, place the other end in your mouth, and blow in and suck out. The light reflex and drum will move. Tympanometry, acoustic reflectometry, uses sound instead of air pressure to determine movement. In suppurative or serous otitis media, the drum is immovable. Serous otitis is a condition with conductive hearing loss. It may be caused by allergies, chronic infections, hypothyroidism, obesity, or anything that contributes to the closure of the eustachian tube. In children with osteopetrosis, the drum is also immovable.

Next, feel and tap the *mastoid* tip of the temporal bone. Note any fluctuation or tenderness; either may indicate mastoiditis. Just behind the mastoid, feel for the postauricular nodes. In children, these are normally about 1 or 2 mm in diameter. Enlarged nodes are characteristic of German measles, nits, or inflammation of the scalp and are usually slightly tender. They are also found in children with measles, roseola, varicella, infectious mononucleosis, leukemia, and tick bites. In this area, you may occasionally feel subcutaneous nodules about 2–5 mm in diameter. These nodules are characteristic of active rheumatic fever.

Estimate *hearing*. In small children, make a sharp noise at the child's ear and note a blinking of the eyes. Each ear is tested separately while you stand outside the direct line of vision of the child. In older children, testing by using the whispered voice at a distance of about 8 feet is sufficient. This is best done by asking the child simple questions or whispering a simple command.

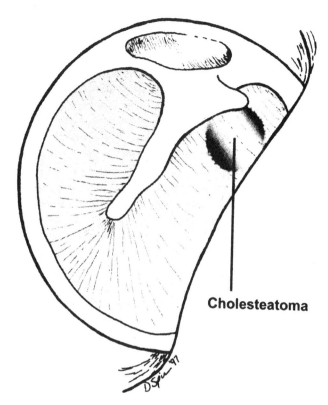

Cholesteatoma

Figure 4-9. A site for cholesteatoma.

Nothing is quite so gratifying as diagnosing impaired hearing in a child who was believed to be mentally delayed.

Loss of hearing can be conductive, neurosensory, or mixed. Most mentally normal children older than 3 years are cooperative enough to be tested with a *tuning fork*. If your hearing is normal, press the tip of the vibrating tuning fork against the mastoid process of the child and then your own. Compare the number of seconds it is heard by both of you. If the child hears it for a shorter time than you, decreased bone conduction is indicated—a sign of neurosensory hearing loss. If the child hears it longer, conductive loss is indicated (Schwabach's test). Compare air and bone conduction in the patient. First place the fork on the mastoid as before and then place it about 1 inch from the child's ear, with approximately equal vibratory stimulus. Normally, air conduction lasts twice as long as bone conduction (Rinne test). Then place the vibrating fork on the middle of the child's forehead and ask in which ear the child hears the sound better. In unilateral conductive deafness, the hearing is better in the unaffected side (Weber test). In unilateral neurosensory deafness, the hearing is better in the affected ear.

Hearing loss may be due simply to a foreign body or cerumen in the canals. Defective hearing may be noted in children with chronic catarrhal otitis media associated with enlarged adenoids or other nasal obstruction, in children who have received dihydrostreptomycin, or in children who have had meningitis, encephalitis, kernicterus, or Hunter syndrome. Congenital deafness is usually idiopathic, but may be found in children whose mothers had rubella during the first trimester of pregnancy. Unilateral deafness may be a sequela of mumps. Deafness associated with syncope may be due to congenital heart lesions (Jervell's and Lange-Nielsen syndrome). Deafness may be associated with hereditary renal disease with hyperprolinemia or with a white forelock and eye abnormalities (Waardenburg syndrome). Pseudodeafness may be observed in psychotic children, especially those with autism, or in children with mental delay. Children with more complicated types of deafness should be referred to an otologist. Hyperacute hearing may occur in children with Tay-Sachs' or lysosomal storage diseases or tetanus.

Children who have received streptomycin or who have nystagmus or an unsteady gait or dizziness (*vertigo*) should have their *vestibular* function tested. The cold caloric test usually suffices. Seat the patient and inject water of 65°F (18°C) into the ear. Nystagmus should appear within 30 seconds, with the fast movement opposite the injected ear. Fast movement toward the injection suggests CNS disease. Repeat the test in the opposite ear. Nystagmus should persist almost equally (for about 1–2 minutes) on each side. Lack of nystagmus suggests lack of labyrinth function or vestibular or brainstem disease. This may be due to streptomycin medication, labyrinthitis, meningitis, or brain tumor, or it may be a sign of benign paroxysmal vertigo. Vertigo with tinnitus and fluctuating hearing loss is characteristic of Ménière disease. Dizziness with progressive hearing loss and facial or corneal numbness occurs with acoustic neuroma. Acute vertigo with nausea and vomiting followed by dysarthria, dysphagia, or unilateral weakness suggests infarct in the medulla with posterior cerebellar or vertebral artery involvement (Wallenberg syndrome). Hiccups may accompany the vertigo. Vertigo with nystagmus that occurs after air pressure is exerted on the drum indicates a fistula, especially with cholesteatoma.

NOSE

Examination of the nose, even a superficial examination, is often neglected, yet it may hold the key to the proper diagnosis.

Note any unusual *shape* of the nose. Because the lower half of the nasal septum is cartilage, fracture or dislocation of the nose is rare in childhood. Deviation is occasionally observed in newborns, possibly due to intrauterine position. The chief cause of flattening of the nose in childhood is cleft palate. With cleft palate or injury the nasal septum is deflected and the nose appears flattened. A saddle-shaped nose is characterized by a low bridge and broad base. This is usually a familial characteristic but also occurs in children with hypertelorism or following perforation of the septum, as in congenital syphilis.

Note *flaring* of the alae nasi. The alae flare with all types of respiratory obstruction or distress but particularly with pneumonia. Flaring of the alae nasi may be seen in children with fevers, acidosis, peritonitis, or any condition or illness causing anoxia.

Next, shine a light up the nose and note the color of the *mucosa*. If you push the tip of the nose upward with the thumb of your left hand and hold the light with your right hand, you can frequently see high into the nose. A speculum is usually not necessary for satisfactory examination of the mucosa or the ostia of the sinuses. If a nasal speculum is desired, use the spring type rather than the otoscope speculum. By placing the large otoscope speculum in the tip of the nose, you can examine the area to the middle meatus. The nasal speculum is preferably used with a head mirror, but satisfactory examination can be performed with a hand light if the patient's head is held firmly. A red, inflamed mucosa indicates infection, including sinusitis. A pale, boggy mucosa may indicate allergy. A swollen grayish mucosa may indicate chronic rhinitis.

Note the character of secretions. Purulent secretions are common with any nasal infection, even the usual upper respiratory infection in its later stages, or may be an early sign of the contagious diseases, particularly measles, pertussis, and poliomyelitis. Purulent secretions from the ostia above or below the middle turbinates indicate sinusitis; pus in the middle meatus suggests involvement of the maxillary, frontal, or anterior ethmoid sinuses; and pus in the superior meatus suggests involvement of the posterior ethmoid or sphenoid sinuses. Patients with discharge and crusting below or on the edges of the alae nasi, particularly with redness of the surrounding skin, usually have infections with β-hemolytic streptococci. Purulent discharges may also be caused by *H. influenzae* or *S. pneumoniae*. Purulent or bloody secretions in infancy may be a sign of secondary syphilis. When due to syphilis, such secretions may occur in children until age 6 months and are usually associated with excoriations of the upper lip.

Watery nasal secretions may indicate allergy, the common cold, foreign bodies high in the nose, illicit drug use or, rarely, skull fracture or perforated encephalocele. Unilateral purulent secretions suggest foreign body, nasal diphtheria, nasal polyps, and sinusitis.

Note *bleeding points* in the nose. They are most commonly found at the lower anterior tip of the septum. Epistaxis is rare in infancy and, if present, may indicate a bleeding dyscrasia. The usual cause of epistaxis, hemoptysis, and hematemesis in children is irritation or injury of the nasal mucosa. Epistaxis is especially common in children with allergic rhinitis. Other less common causes of epistaxis include nasal infections (particularly diphtheria); typhoid fever; leukemia; rheumatic fever; foreign body; and congestion due to any cause such as congenital heart disease. Occasionally, epistaxis in childhood is caused by late syphilis, elevated blood pressure due to any cause, or any of the anemias or bleeding diseases. Bleeding after skull injury may be due to local nasal injury or to skull fracture. Rarely, a bleeding telangiectasis is noted in the mucosa and may be the cardinal sign of familial telangiectasia. Epistaxis may be the only physical sign of hereditary hemorrhagic thrombasthenia, one of the bleeding diseases.

Note the child's ability to get air through the nose. Infection, foreign body, vasomotor rhinitis, tumor, polyp, or a badly deviated septum are the usual causes of inability to breathe through the nose. Newborns with bilateral choanal atresia are unable to get air through the nostrils and often appear to be choking. In the older child, large adenoids, even if uninfected, may cause nasal obstruction with a typical adenoid facies. Obstruction with recurrent epistaxis, especially in teenage boys, suggests angiofibroma.

An unusually large nasal airway with dry crusting is occasionally noted. This may be a sign of atrophic rhinitis, which occurs in older children or adults. A malodorous nasal discharge may be present.

In the older child, examine the nasal *septum*. Perforation may be due to injury of the nasal septum, foreign body, syphilis, tuberculosis, or sniffing of illicit drugs.

Occasionally *polyps* or *tumors* may occlude one nostril or even protrude from the nose. Polyps frequently occur with allergy, but may be a manifestation of chronic infection, cystic fibrosis, or generalized polyposis. An encephalocele may protrude through the cribriform plate and appear to be a polyp. If you observe a membrane in the nose preceded by bleeding, consider diphtheria until this diagnosis can be eliminated.

Percuss the sinus areas for evidence of pain as previously described. Olfactory nerve tests are generally not performed in childhood. Anosmia is a sign of Kallmann's syndrome, zinc deficiency, and chronic nasal infection.

MOUTH AND THROAT

Defer examination of the mouth and throat until the end of the examination in young children. For you to see the posterior pharynx and particularly the epiglottis during gagging, the child must be sitting and cooperative or adequately restrained when the depressor is finally placed far in the mouth. If the mother or an assistant is present, the child can sit on that person's lap. Ask the mother or assistant to hold both the child's wrists with one hand and the forehead with the other (Fig. 4-10). Examine the external structures first.

Around the mouth, note *circumoral pallor*. With circumoral pallor, the immediate area around the mouth appears white, and the strip just below the nose, the surface of the cheeks, and the lower chin are red. This appearance may occur with any febrile disease, but it is particularly noted in children who have just exercised or who have scarlet or rheumatic fever or hypoglycemia. Even in infants with seborrheic dermatitis and eczema, this pale area usually remains free of lesions, although the remainder of the cheeks may be covered with scales.

Inspect the *lips*. Asymmetry of the mouth with twisting of the lips to one side occurs with facial nerve or trigeminal nerve paralysis. Cleft lip, usually on the left side, is a congenital anomaly. Note extent and location of the cleft. Lip pits may appear as isolated deformities or may be associated with other anomalies.

Slight *fissures* of the lips (cheilitis) occur in children exposed to wind and sun and in children with Kawasaki disease. Rhagades are deep fissures or their resultant scars extending from the nose to the lips and extending outward from the lips. They are characteristic of congenital syphilis. Deep painful fis-

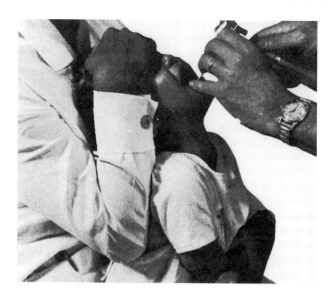

Figure 4-10. Restraint of patient in sitting position to examine posterior pharynx and epiglottis.

sures radiating from the ends of the lips (cheilosis) are apparent in children with numerous nutritional disturbances, particularly riboflavin and other B vitamin, protein, or iron deficiencies, or with *Candida* and other infections. Excoriation of the upper lip is common in young children with simple upper respiratory infections. Painful ulcers on the lips and adjacent tissues are characteristic of erythema multiforme, but if chronic may be due to squamous cell carcinoma.

Vesicles and pustules appear on the lips in older children, especially after upper respiratory infections. "Cold sores" (herpes simplex) are vesicles on an inflamed base and usually burn or itch. Bacterial infections are detected as ordinary pustules. Retention cysts, usually single, occur on the lip and appear as small protrusions containing clear fluid.

Note the *color* of the lips. The normal pink of white children and gray of black children is replaced by a pale mucosa when anemia is present. Gray cyanosis is seen with most congenital heart lesions, methemoglobinemia, anoxia, and bizarre poisons. Deep-purple lips are seen with severe congenital heart disease. Cherry-red lips are characteristically seen in infants and children with acidosis and are frequently due to aspirin poisoning or diabetes in older children and in patients with carbon monoxide poisoning. With many poisons, the child's lips may appear red although the body is pallid. Telangiectases in the lips may herald Rendu-Osler-Weber syndrome (familial telangiectasia).

The lips may be grossly *swollen* due to insect bites, local infection or injury, angioneurotic edema, or massive generalized edema.

Note unusual *odors* from the mouth which may suggest an organic acidemia (see Chapter 3). The sweetish odor of acetone is common in dehydrated or malnourished children but may indicate diabetic acidosis as in adults. Children with diphtheria exude a mouselike odor. Children with typhoid fever may exude an odor similar to that of decaying tissue. An ammoniacal odor occurs in children with uremia. Halitosis (bad breath) occurs in children with many varied states, including poor local hygiene, local or systemic infections, sinusitis, and mouth breathing.

It is useless to ask a child aged less than 6 or 7 years if the throat hurts, since even with acute pharyngitis or tonsillitis, the child usually has no pain. If pain is present in younger children, it more commonly indicates the presence of epiglottitis or laryngitis or occasionally abscess, diphtheria, or scarlatina.

Good lighting, preferably daylight, is necessary for further examination. Become accustomed to the use of one type of light, either daylight or electric. To grasp well what you see, develop the ability to anticipate the normal throat structures and to retain an afterimage of the abnormalities seen. With practice, you will learn to prolong the gag, so that the structures can be more carefully visualized.

Most patients will open their mouths when asked to do so. Inability of a child to open the mouth is generally only voluntary and not true inability. Ask the child to breathe rapidly through the mouth or to say "No", "Ah", or "Eh". If the child makes the sound loud enough, the mouth opens wide. True inability to open the mouth occurs with tetanus (trismus), tetany, infections in the tissues surrounding the mouth, peritonsillar abscess, dislocation of the temporomandibular joint and, occasionally, parotitis. In rheumatic fever or rheumatoid arthritis, the swollen temporomandibular joint will sometimes prevent the patient from opening the mouth. Ankylosis of the joint may occur secondary to birth injury to the joint. Temporomandibular joint involvement can frequently be recognized not only by the apparent inability to move the joint, but also by obvious asymmetry of the face. Trismus may also occur in children with infantile Gaucher disease, brain tumor, or encephalitis, and it is common in children who receive phenothiazine derivatives.

If the child does not open the mouth after suggestion, tell the child that examination of the throat is not really painful but may be uncomfortable and that the examination will take "only a second." If the child is 18 months of age or older, attempting to have the child open the mouth voluntarily is worthwhile. One device is to ask if the child would like to examine a relative (brother, sister, or cousin) after leaving. Most children say "Yes." Give the child a tongue blade and say: "I'll show you how to do it. First you have your brother open his mouth wide. Then you look at his teeth, then you look high, and then you look low." Even though a gag is elicited, most children are not very angry.

If this suggestion fails, tell the child to show the teeth. Then attempt to place the tongue blade on the anterior part of the tongue for a view of the tongue and palate. With the blade in this position, the child is not uncomfortable and usually does not resist patient examination. If the child resists by closing the mouth and gritting the teeth, carefully and firmly restrain the child.

Place the tongue blade gently between the lips to the posterior teeth and push the mucosa away from the teeth to obtain an adequate view of the teeth, gums, and mucosa. Use small tongue blades for small children. If mouth lesions are suspected, it is frequently less painful if the tongue blade is moistened before it is inserted. Patiently, push the blade between the teeth toward the pharynx. Insert the blade with a slightly downward motion so that the tongue is pushed forward and the base of the tongue downward. Suddenly, the child will gag, the mouth will open, and in that instant, observe all the structures inside the mouth. At no time should the nose be pinched closed (see Fig. 4-9). Because the child almost immediately resists further manipulation, this part of the examination should be performed expeditiously, and you should know exactly what you wish to learn before causing the gag.

The first area that presents with the gag is the *epiglottis*, located at the base of the tongue. Note swelling and color. A swollen red epiglottis is apparent in some children with laryngotracheobronchitis, especially when it is due to *H. influenzae*, and may obstruct respiration. With viral infections and allergy, the epiglottis is swollen and pale. Either a swollen red or swollen pale epiglottitis may represent a respiratory emergency. A congenitally large epiglottis or ulcers of the epiglottis may be noted. Lack of gag may be due to ninth or tenth nerve injury and is sometimes seen in patients with bulimia.

Next inspect the *uvula*. A very long uvula is congenital and may cause gagging or coughing. Occasionally, the uvula is congenitally bifid and may be associated with a submucous cleft of the palate. It may be absent, having been accidentally removed during tonsillectomy. Note motion of the uvula and soft palate as the patient is gagged or told to say "Ah." Paralysis of the soft palate or uvula or absence of the gag reflex is an early sign of poliomyelitis and diphtheria, but is also noted in disorders involving the glossopharyngeal or vagus nerves or conditions with masses behind the palate. Limited motion of the soft palate may be caused by hypertrophied, infected adenoids. A translucent membrane in the midline of the soft palate indicates lack of continuity of muscles and may be a sign of palatopharyngeal incompetence.

Look at the posterior *pharynx* for lymphoid hyperplasia, color, postnasal drip, membrane, edema, exudate, abscess, and vesicles. Lymphoid hyperplasia is evident with any infection of the area. A red, inflamed pharynx is characteristic of any type of acute pharyngitis, but there are no good local signs to distinguish bacterial from nonbacterial pharyngitis. A pale, puffy mucosa indicates edema. Vesicles on the posterior pharynx, anterior pillars, or uvula surrounded by erythema of 3–6 mm are a sign of herpangina due to Coxsackie virus A infection. These vesicles ulcerate, and small ulcers may remain for 2–3 weeks. Small maculopapules on the posterior pharynx are also seen in other respiratory viral diseases.

Profuse postnasal drip indicates infection in the nose, nasopharynx, or sinuses and may cause a foul odor. A white membrane over the tonsils or posterior pharynx is evident in children with diphtheria; other bacterial infections, particularly Vincent's angina and β-hemolytic streptococcal infection;

infectious mononucleosis; agranulocytosis; and leukemia. In diphtheria, the mouth smells "mousy," and the membrane pulls away with bleeding. The membrane in diphtheria is usually more confluent than in the other infections and spreads to cover more of the uvula and posterior pharynx. Indeed, a confluent membrane involving the uvula or posterior pharynx should be considered diphtheritic until proved otherwise.

The pharynx or throat is separated from the mouth by the anterior and posterior pillars. The palatine (faucial) *tonsils* are located between these pillars. Note size of the tonsils. Like all lymphoid tissue, tonsils are much larger during early childhood than later; therefore, you should not make statements regarding enlargement of tonsils in childhood until you have examined many normal tonsils or until obstruction of the airway is obvious.

Crypts in the tonsillar tissue may indicate past infection; pus in the tonsils and peritonsillar abscesses indicate acute infections. The tonsils appear to be pushed backward or forward and the uvula may be displaced with peritonsillar abscesses. Peritonsillar abscesses occur more often in older children and are usually due to streptococcus infections.

In infants aged less than 2 years, erythema of the tonsils usually occurs with bacterial infections, especially streptococci, pneumococci, and *H. influenzae*. Purulent exudate or membrane suggests the presence of viral infections. In children aged more than 2 years, some attempt can be made to distinguish bacterial from viral tonsillitis, although obtaining cultures of the nasopharynx is usually necessary. Yellow or grayish-white follicles are usually due to bacteria. Vesicles, nodules, punched-out ulcers, scanty or streaky membranes, and patchy gray, white, or yellow membranes usually indicate viral infection. A coalescent white membrane occurs with *Candida* infections. A bluish-gray membrane with ulceration is more common in children with agranulocytosis or other severe underlying hematologic disorders.

Tuberculosis and tumors may also cause enlargement of the tonsils. Definite unilateral enlargement of the tonsillar area is common with diseases such as Vincent infection, diphtheria, and lymphoma. Enlarged, lobulated, red-orange tonsils have been reported in association with accumulation of cholesterol esters (Tangier disease).

Collections of movable mucus and pus may be noted in the posterior pharynx. This is usually postnasal drip and may be caused by sinusitis or infected adenoids.

Outpouching of the posterior pharyngeal wall is characteristic of retropharyngeal abscess. Examination of the retropharynx with a finger is usually necessary only if an abscess or submucous cleft is suspected. Retropharyngeal abscesses usually occur in children in the first 2 years of life; they are felt as unilateral soft masses in infants who are usually quite ill and have noisy respirations and, occasionally, retracted necks.

Single ulcers without generalized symptoms are canker sores. A recurrent type of canker sore may occur with allergy. Sudden swelling of any part of the buccal mucosa also occurs with allergy.

Other types of stomatitis occurring on the mucosa include vesicles of chickenpox, mucous patches of early congenital syphilis, and general inflammation with vesicles of the erythroderma desquamativum syndromes.

Most children aged 2 1/2 years or older will open the mouth, and the posterior pharynx can be visualized. Examine the throat at this time. Do not restrain patients unless they move. In older children, if you push down first one side of the tongue and then the other, visualizing all the mouth and throat is sometimes easier. Frequently, if the patient sticks the tongue out and breathes deeply, the tongue blade need not be used.

Usually, little *salivary secretion* is seen in infants until 3 months of age. Absence of salivation may indicate dehydration, fever, Mikulicz syndrome, botulism, atropine ingestion, or congenital ectodermal dysplasia. Drooling or collection of saliva in the mouth is normal in children until 2 years of age and persists in those with swallowing difficulty and injury to the glossopharyngeal (IX) or vagal (X) nerves or with encephalitis or myasthenia. Gag reflex may be decreased.

Thick mucoid secretions are frequently evident after tracheal irritation. Unswallowed saliva or excess mucoid secretions are noted in newborns with tracheoesophageal fistula, probably due to aspirated gastric secretions with secondary tracheal irritation.

Note excessive salivation or drooling. A child aged 2–5 years who is in respiratory distress, sitting up, and drooling should first be considered to have epiglottitis. If you do suspect epiglottitis, DO NOT advance the tongue blade.

Excessive Salivation

Teething	Caustic exposure
Caries	Mental delay
Mouth infection	Gingivostomatitis
Mercury poison	Phosphate poison
Familial dysautonomia	Acrodynia
Salivary gland infections	Smokeless tobacco

Note inflammation, color, swelling, and distortions of the *gums*. Children with gingivitis have redness, swelling, and tenderness of the gums. Inflammation of the gingiva may indicate the presence of a systemic disease or vitamin C deficiency, or it may occur in mouth breathers or in children with erupting teeth, poor mouth hygiene, or poor dental care. Swelling or small cysts on the hard palate or gums in infants may be a sign of pneumococcal sepsis.

In children with teeth, a black line along the margin of the gum may signify heavy metal poisoning. However, a melanotic line of the gums themselves is found in normal black infants. The gums near the teeth are purple and bleed easily in children with scurvy, in children with other bleeding diseases such as leukemia or chronic leukopenia, in children with poor oral hygiene, and sometimes in apparently normal children. The gums in children with herpetic stomatitis appear to be painted with a bright red pencil and are swollen and tender. Generalized hypertrophy of the gums is seen in mouth breathers, in children receiving phenytoin who have phenytoin sensitivity, in children with hereditary gingival fibromatosis, and in many vitamin deficiency states. Pinpoint inflamed elevations from which pus can be expressed with the tongue depressor are characteristic of abscess of the tooth root.

In young infants, epithelial pearls or retention cysts are found in or near the midline of the gums. These cysts have no clinical significance and usually disappear spontaneously when the infant is 2–3 months of age. Asymptomatic white patches on the cheeks or lips in older children may represent ectopic sebaceous glands (Fordyce spots).

Next, inspect the *buccal mucosa*. In young infants, look especially for thrush, small white patches that bleed when scraped off or rubbed. Thrush in a newborn may result from maternal infection. It also occurs in debilitated children or in children with hypoparathyroidism and after prolonged antibiotic use. Fixed white patches that do not rub off are leukoplakia or lichen planus. Patches that scrape off are usually due to milk or other ingested white food. Bluish-white scattered spots about the size of a grain of sand on the buccal mucosa at the level of the lower teeth and within the lower lip are characteristic of Koplik spots. These spots usually indicate measles. Red spots 1–3 mm in diameter over the buccal mucosa and palate are characteristic of Forschheimer sign, frequently an early indication of German measles. Vesicles on the buccal mucosa, especially if surrounded by a red line, are usually due to herpes simplex. If on the posterior pharynx, similar vesicles usually indicate herpangina due to Coxsackie virus infection. Pale red spots may cover the buccal mucosa in measles and other viral diseases and are the enanthems of the diseases with skin exanthems. Painful mouth ulcers may be aphthous ulcers of unknown cause.

Painful Mouth Ulcers

Unknown causes	Erythema multiforme
Immune deficiency	Leukemia
Folic acid deficiency	Neutropenia
Vitamin B_{12} deficiency	Inflammatory bowel disease (e.g., Crohn disease)
Niacin or tryptophan deficiency	Diphtheria

Veins on the buccal mucosa are ordinarily not apparent. Visible or dilated veins on the buccal mucosa or tongue may be a sign of cyanosis or may indicate cardiac failure or local vascular obstruction.

View the *tongue*. Normally, the dorsal surface of the tongue is coated with conical filiform papillae. The circumvallate papillae form a V on the posterior third of the tongue. Coating may signify mouth breathing or lack of motion of the tongue caused by debility in severe disease. Dry tongue is a sign of general dehydration. Unilateral atrophy of the tongue may be due to injury of the hypoglossal nerve.

Large red *papillae* resembling a strawberry or raspberry are seen with scarlet fever. On the tip and sides are profusion of red dots about 1 mm in diameter, the fungiform papillae. A uniformly smooth tongue with no apparent fungiform papillae is a sign of familial dysautonomia. Black tongue may be congenital but has been described as a low-grade infection subsequent to penicillin administration or chickenpox. It also occurs in mouth bleeders, as in patients with hemophilia (see box).

Tongue	
White patches	Thrush, milk
Red, sore	Riboflavin deficiency
	Niacin deficiency
	Anemia
Melanotic pigment	Adrenal insufficiency
	Acanthosis nigricans
	Cachexia
	Neurofibromatosis
	Pellagra
Melanotic patches	Polyposis (Peutz syndrome)
Black	Congenital, oral antibiotic
	Chicken pox
	Mouth bleeders
Bright red	Kawasaki disease
Hairy	Debility, human immunodeficiency syndrome
Petechiae	Platelet abnormal
	Sexual abuse

Geographic tongue consists of gray, irregular areas of the tongue and is usually due to unknown benign cause, but it may be related to febrile states or to allergy. Mentally delayed children have deep furrows in the tongue due to biting of the protruding tongue. However, furrowed tongue is most commonly a congenital characteristic. Scars on the tongue may be due to previous convulsions.

Macroglossia (large tongue) is usually congenital and is a cardinal sign of Beckwith-Weideman syndrome. It may be an early sign of hypothyroidism or mucopolysaccharidosis or be due to a lymphangioma, cyst, or hemangioma. In patients who let the tongue protrude, the tongue may appear large. Protrusion of the tongue may also be due to a tumor or thyroglossal duct cyst at the base of the tongue.

Tongue-tie is caused by a very short frenum. If the tongue tip of an infant does not interfere with feeding or if an older child can elevate the tip to produce the sounds of *t,d,n* and *l,* the condition does not exist. A torn frenulum may be due to child abuse. Cysts or ranulae are occasionally seen in the floor of the mouth near the frenum.

Note *tremor* of the tongue as it protrudes. Fine tremor is seen with chorea, hyperthyroidism, and amyotonia congenita. Gross tremor may be seen in children with cerebral palsy. Fibrillations (slow undulating movements) indicate completely denervated muscle and may be an early sign of spinal muscular atrophy (Werdnig-Hoffmann disease).

Paralysis of the tongue may be noted. The tongue protrudes toward the involved side in patients with hypoglossal nerve lesions.

With the tongue depressor still on the anterior half of the child's tongue, inspect the hard *palate*. Note color of the palate. You may detect jaundice. Petechiae on the palate are usually due to any condition causing pharyngitis but may be due to other diseases that cause petechiae on the skin or elsewhere.

Look for congenital *cleft palate*. Note if the cleft involves only the hard palate, the soft palate, or the uvula and distinguish it from the rare condition of palatal perforation. Perforation of the palate occurs after age 2 years in those who have congenital syphilis. High, arched palates are usually seen in mouth breathers but are also seen in children with arachnodactyly and many other congenital disorders. Hypertrophy of the bone in the midline of the palate (torus palatinus) is usually an anomaly of little significance.

Inspect the *teeth* for number, caries, and type of occlusion. Compare the number of teeth present with the averages for age (Table 4-1). Occasionally a tooth will be seen in a newborn. Delayed appearance of the deciduous teeth (e.g., after 1 year of age) may be normal, especially in obese children, or may indicate cretinism, rickets, congenital syphilis, or Down syndrome. Absence of teeth is seen with congenital ectodermal dysplasia. Loss of teeth is seen in children with metabolic diseases such as acrodynia, xanthomatosis, histiocytosis, cherubism, gingivitis, and low-phosphatase rickets. In children who grind their teeth the edges of the teeth are usually flattened. The usual causes of tooth grinding (bruxism) are psychologic difficulties, mental delay, tiredness, and local irritation.

Malocclusion may occur without obvious cause or after premature loss or prolonged retention of deciduous teeth. It may be a family characteristic, and it also occurs in children with mouth breathing, cleft palate, micrognathia, or prognathism. One cause of malocclusion of permanent teeth is persistent thumbsucking after 6 years of age.

Table 4-1. *Chronology of tooth eruption*

Primary		Secondary	
Maxillary			
Central incisor	7½ mo	Central incisor	7–8 yr
Lateral incisor	9 mo	Lateral incisor	8–9 yr
Cuspid	18 mo	Cuspid	11–12 yr
First molar	14 mo	First bicuspid	10–11 yr
Second molar	24 mo	Second bicuspid	10–12 yr
		First molar	6–7 yr
		Second molar	12–13 yr
		Third molar	17–21 yr
Mandibular			
Central incisor	6 mo	Central incisor	6–7 yr
Lateral incisor	7 mo	Lateral incisor	7–8 yr
Cuspid	16 mo	Cuspid	9–10 yr
First molar	12 mo	First bicuspid	11–12 yr
Second molar	20 mo	Second bicuspid	11–12 yr
		First molar	6–7 yr
		Second molar	11–13 yr
		Third molar	17–21 yr

Dental *caries*, due to bacterial decay and disintegration of tooth substance, are difficult to detect without special instruments until cavitation occurs. Disintegration of the enamel may be detected with a sharp instrument, especially if tooth pain is present. The number of caries is decreased in children with Down syndrome, fructose intolerance, and sucrose intolerance and is increased in children with chronic infection, including human immunodeficiency virus (HIV).

Poor tooth formation may be evident in systemic diseases such as hypocalcemia, congenital lues, hypoparathyroidism, severe infections, and nutritional disturbances, including rickets and nephrosis. Enamel formation in primary teeth is defective in children with prenatal infections or cerebral palsy. Older children or adolescents with bulimia may have defective posterior incisors.

Green or black teeth may be found after iron ingestion or after death of the tooth. Green teeth are also seen in children who had severe jaundice at birth. Red teeth are sometimes seen in those with porphyria. Brown teeth may be due to congenital defect in tooth formation. Mottled, pitted teeth may be seen after excess fluoride ingestion and some years after treatment with tetracycline. The back of the teeth may be eroded in those with bulimia. Centrally notched, peg-shaped permanent teeth (Hutchinson teeth) may occur in children with congenital syphilis. Mulberrylike 6-year molars occur in normal children but may also indicate congenital syphilis.

After you examine the throat, break the tongue depressor in front of the child and throw it away so that the child knows that this part of the examination has ended.

Vomiting is actually a symptom. However, when vomiting occurs, note the nature of the vomitus and save the vomitus if physical and chemical examinations are desired. Vomiting in newborns may have special significance.

Overfeeding, food intolerance, and improper handling of the infant are the usual causes of vomiting during infancy. However, vomiting of recently ingested food in children may be an early sign of infection in the intestinal tract or elsewhere. A common form of severe vomiting occurs in children 2–12 years of age; it occurs periodically, is probably due to a combination of psychogenic factors and lability of ketone-producing mechanisms, and is termed *cyclic vomiting*. Vomiting associated with nausea and occurring before breakfast may indicate hypoglycemia. Vomiting without nausea or vomiting of liquids but not solids, especially in the early morning, may be a sign of brain tumor.

Vomiting

Cough	Gastroesophageal reflux
Increased intracranial pressure	Migraine
Brain tumor	Poison (e.g., lead)
Food allergy	Medications
Enteritis	Parenteral infections
Chalasia	Psychogenic
Metabolic diseases	Abdominal epilepsy

In infants, forceful vomiting, especially of curdled milk free of bile staining, may be a sign of pylorospasm or pyloric stenosis but may also be the presenting sign of imperforate hymen. Vomitus containing bile may indicate duodenal or jejunal obstruction, whereas fecal vomiting is more common in children with lower intestinal obstruction, ileus, or peritonitis.

Bloody vomitus is most commonly due to swallowed blood from the nose and upper respiratory tract or from the mother's fissured nipple in a breast-fed infant. It is also seen in children with hemorrhagic diseases including Henoch-Schoenlein purpura, after the ingestion of foreign body or poisons, and after severe vomiting from any cause. Occasionally, bloody vomitus is seen in children with gastric, duodenal, or esophageal ulcers, anomalies of the portal vein, or cirrhosis of the liver with esophageal varices.

LARYNX

Note the *voice* or *cry* for hoarseness or stridor. Stridor is due to obstruction in the airway. In the first 3 years of life, it is considered an emergency until cause is found. Inspiratory stridor generally indicates an extrathoracic lesion, and expiratory stridor occurs with an intrathoracic obstruction.

Expiratory Stridor

Subglottic edema	Asthma
Subglottic mass	Cystic fibrosis
Vascular ring	Tracheomalacia
Bronchopulmonary dysplasia	Bronchomalacia

If the obstruction is so severe that the airway cannot dilate, the stridor will be both inspiratory and expiratory. Low-pitched stridor, especially if accompanied by salivation or snoring, indicates inflammation in the supraglottic area. The cry or voice is muffled, and dysphagia may be present. Snoring indicates upper airway obstruction, such as large tonsils or adenoids or a mass at the base of the tongue. During inspiration with glottic obstruction, crowing is high-pitched, the voice is hoarse or aphonic, and pain is present. During inspiration with subglottic inflammation or obstruction or with vocal cord paralysis, high-pitched stridor with a weak cry and little hoarseness occurs.

Stridor associated with wheezing occurs with intrathoracic or extrathoracic lesions such as tracheal inflammation (croup), in which it is both inspiratory and expiratory. A low-pitched fluttering sound that is best heard over the larynx is characteristic of laryngomalacia. Grunting with respiratory illness may be due to chest pain or may be a physiologic response to maintain increased airway pressure during expiration.

Hoarseness or Stridor

Laryngitis	Shouting
Trancheitis	Hypothyroid
Allergy	Tetanus
Croup	Gaucher's disease
Retropharyngeal abscess	Lysosomal storage
Laryngeal foreign body	Vascular ring

Hoarseness due to infection is more common in viral laryngitis or laryngitis due to *H. influenzae* than in infection due to streptococci. Cretins have a low raucous cry and children with de Lange's syndrome emit a growl. Infants with severe gastrointestinal disturbances such as intussusception and peritonitis have a sharp whining cry. Some children with a rare chromosome abnormality involving a deletion of material from chromosome 5 emit a catlike cry (cri-du-chat syndrome). Nasal speech may occur in children with chronic upper respiratory infection, enlarged adenoids, deafness, and neurogenic or anatomic velopharyngeal incompetence such as in children with cleft palate.

Laryngoscopy is not performed in the routine examination. Unless good presumptive cause of the hoarseness exists, laryngoscopy is necessary. It is best performed in young children with an electric laryngoscope of small or medium size with good batteries and light. The child should be placed in a supine position and should have an empty stomach to obviate aspiration of vomitus during manipulation. The head is held with the neck partly flexed by the mother. The child's tongue is held, and the laryngoscope is slowly inserted along the tongue to the base. Visualize the posterior pharynx and epiglottis and note their status. A redundant large epiglottis may be seen when it obstructs the airway.

Pass the laryngoscope over the epiglottis and pull the handle up slightly toward the patient's head until you see the larynx. You may note laryngeal spasm, edema, paralysis, stenosis, redundancy, and tumors. You may also see thyroglossal duct cysts at the base of the tongue and the subglottic area if the larynx is normal.

In older children who can cooperate, indirect laryngoscopy is less traumatic. Seat the patient, warm the mirror, grasp the tongue, and pass the mirror back to rest on the anterior surface of the uvula, pushing it upward and backward. With good lighting, you can see the larynx. The cords are best seen if you tell the patient to say "eeee." This is the best diagnostic method for examination of the larynx when it can be used. It is particularly useful in problems of laryngeal motility and should precede direct laryngoscopy if possible.

Listen to the young child *speak*. The child should speak a word or two at 1 year of age and should put two- to three-word sentences together at 2 years of age. Speech should be almost completely intelligible by 4 years of age. In children who are hearing or visually impaired or mentally delayed or who have neurologic or physical abnormalities of the vocalizing apparatus, speech is delayed or limited. In older children, note specific speech defects such as lisping or stuttering. Adolescent males and children with adrenogenital syndrome and sexual precocity of other types have a deep voice. Children with large adenoids, sinusitis, or palatal paralysis have a nasal voice. Slurred indistinct speech with clicking produced by the tongue forcibly hitting the hard palate occurs in chorea. Aphonia with ability to whisper may indicate hysteria.

NECK

Examination of the neck takes 1 to 2 seconds but may help in the diagnosis of many diseases. The patient should be lying flat on the back or sitting.

First, note the *size* of the neck. The neck normally appears short during infancy and lengthens at about 3–4 years of age. Children with platybasia, cretinism, or Morquio, Hurler, and Klippel-Feil syndromes have a short neck. *Webbing* of the neck is sometimes noted in children with gonadal dysgenesis or as an isolated anomaly. Marked *edema* of the neck is noted in children with local infections, cellulitis, diphtheria, other infections of the mouth, mumps, obstruction of the superior vena cava, and any of the causes of generalized edema.

Next, palpate the anterior and posterior cervical triangles for *lymph nodes* (described in Chapter 3). Observe or palpate other *masses* in the neck. Enlarged parotids usually extend down into the neck. Cystic masses in the midline high in the neck that are freely movable and move upward when the patient swallows may be thyroglossal duct cysts. Pulling the tongue forward causes these cystic areas to move. Fistula may accompany the cyst. Midline cystlike masses that do not move freely may be lingual thyroid cysts, sebaceous cysts, lipomas, or dermoids. Diffuse swelling of the neck with nonpitting edema (bull neck) is seen in children with severe diphtheria.

Next palpate the *sternocleidomastoid muscle*. A mass in the lower third of the sternocleidomastoid muscle generally indicates congenital torticollis. Torticollis without abnormality in the muscle may be associated with gastroesophageal reflux and neuroblastoma. Oval, cystic, smooth, moderately movable masses near the upper third of the muscle are usually due to branchial cysts and may be associated with fistula or may be attached to the skin, with a small dimple. These are almost always anterior to the sternocleidomastoid muscle. Cystic hygroma, which is usually posterior and above either clavicle, and hemangioma are easily compressible. Transilluminate for cystic hygroma or lymphangioma. Other masses include dermoids, neurofibroma, ectopic thyroid, and lipoma. Hard masses suggest Hodgkin disease; lymphosarcoma, rhabdomyosarcoma, or other sarcomas; and metastatic disease, neuroblastoma, and salivary or other malignancies. The callus of a fractured clavicle may be felt as a hard mass.

Next, palpate the *trachea*, feeling first the most anterior parts with one finger and then proceeding down both sides simultaneously with your thumb and index finger. The trachea should be slightly to the right of the midline. Any further deviation in either direction indicates mediastinal shift due to atelectasis (especially due to foreign body), effusion, pneumothorax, or tumor in the chest or neck. A palpatory *thud* (or audible slap) may be felt or heard over the trachea and may indicate the presence of a foreign body free in the trachea.

Next, feel just below the thyroid cartilage for the *thyroid* isthmus and for both lobes of the thyroid just lateral to the thyroid cartilage. The thyroid in younger children can be felt while the child is lying supine. Place your thumb on one side and your index and second fingers on the opposite side of the thyroid cartilage. In older children, it may be easier to palpate the thyroid from behind, with two fingers of each hand placed on both sides of the thyroid cartilage. The thyroid is observed or is felt to move upward when the patient swallows. Note size, shape, position, mobility, and tenderness.

Thyroid enlargement may be due to hyperactive thyroid, malignancy, or goiter. A smooth, enlarged thyroid mass indicates thyroid hyperplasia. Nodules in the thyroid are usually adenomatous and may be malignant. Enlarged tender thyroid indicates early thyroiditis. A woody feel is characteristic of Hashimoto thyroiditis. Unilateral tenderness subsequent to tonsillitis may be due to thrombophlebitis of the internal jugular vein.

Goiter with hypothyroidism may be due to antithyroid drugs or foods, Hashimoto thyroiditis, enzymatic defect in hormone synthesis, or a deficit in iodine. Hypothyroidism without goiter may be hereditary, congenital, or familial or may be due to pituitary disease, sarcoid, or xanthomatosis.

Observe the *vessels* of the neck. Enlarged veins or abnormal venous pulsations may be due to increased venous pressure, which may be caused by heart failure, pericarditis, or masses in the mediastinum. Pulsation of the carotids may sometimes be observed in children, usually after exercise or emotional upset, but may indicate aortic insufficiency, anemia, hypertension, or patent ductus arteriosus. Venous pulsations in the neck in a child who is upright are always abnormal. In contrast to arterial pulsation, venous pulsations are obliterated by light jugular compression. Distended neck veins do not occur in patients with severe liver disease unless heart disease is also present. When heart failure is suspected, press on the liver. If the jugular veins become prominent (the hepatojugular reflex), failure is present. This sign may be misleading in very young children because they perform Valsalva maneuver on abdominal pressure, making the jugular veins stand out. If the jugular veins do not fill on liver pressure, the venous system is not patent. This is a sign of hepatic vein thrombosis (Budd-Chiari syndrome). Unilateral distension suggests an intrathoracic abnormality. Bulging and collapse with expiration and inspiration indicate wide swings in intrathoracic pressure during respiration.

Note two small venous pulse waves: the *A* wave coincides with right atrial contraction, and the *V* wave coincides with right ventricular contraction. A prominent *A* wave occurs in patients with cor pulmonale, tricuspid stenosis or atresia, and pulmonary stenosis or hypertension. Patients with auricular fibrillation do not manifest *A* waves. The *V* wave is prominent in patients with tricuspid insufficiency.

Venous pressure can be fairly accurately determined by measuring the distance from the upper border of the clavicle to the upper level of venous distention in the neck with the child in the sitting position.

The *carotid sinus* may be massaged in children who have histories indicative of possible heart block. Perform such massage only with the stethoscope on the chest. The carotid sinus is best reached by following the carotid artery up to the angle of the jaw and covering the whole area with your thumb. Massaging this area, one side at a time, normally slows the heart 10–20 beats per minute. A greater decrease in rate indicates abnormal carotid sensitivity, a rare cause of syncope.

Auscultate the neck with the bell stethoscope. Murmurs may be heard particularly over the carotid area, but also elsewhere in the neck, and are frequently transmitted from the heart with organic disease. Distinguish the benign venous hum near the carotids from an organic murmur by absence of a similar sound over the heart. To-and-fro bruits may be heard over an enlarged thyroid. Bruits over the carotid artery may be due to increased vascular flow, as noted in persons with hyperthyroidism, anemia, or arteriovenous fistula. Bruits from aortic stenosis murmurs are heard bilaterally low in the middle part of the neck or at the angles of the jaw, which are the carotid areas. Those of vascular insufficiency are usually higher and unilateral. Other sounds in the neck may indicate other vascular anomalies. Listen on each side high along the anterior border of the sternocleidomastoid muscle, the midneck, the lower neck, and the supraclavicular space. Transmitted sounds from the trachea may obliterate these sounds, except during the clear interval between inspiration and expiration.

Finally, note *motion*. First ask the patient to touch the chest with the chin and to turn the head from side to side. If the patient is unable to do this, raise the head from the pillow with one hand and turn the patient's head from side to side. Resistance to flexion of the neck (stiff neck) is characteristic of meningitis or meningeal irritation; in debilitated children with these diseases, the neck may remain supple.

Stiff neck may also be noted with the viral encephalitides, tetanus, lead poisoning, meningismus, and rheumatoid arthritis. It is noted in pharyngitis, cervical adenitis, retropharyngeal abscess, subluxation of the cervical vertebrae due to retropharyngeal or peritonsillar abscess, herniation of the cerebellar tonsils with increased intracranial pressure, and degenerative nervous system diseases as part of their generalized hypertonia. Brudzinski sign, obtained by flexing the neck and noting flexion at the hip, knee, or ankle, is a similar indication of CNS irritation. Episodic tonic axial extension and lateral flexion of the head may be associated with gastroesophageal reflux or hiatus hernia (Sandifer syndrome).

Hyperextension of the neck (*opisthotonos*) is due to any of the causes of stiff neck of a more severe degree. It occurs with respiratory tract obstruction and also in children with cerebral palsy or kernicterus. It is noted periodically in all normal infants or in infants with breath-holding spells. Recurrent hyperextension to lessen obstruction from tracheal compression strongly suggests vascular ring. True opisthotonos, which is a rigid prolonged hyperextension of the spine, usually denotes a completely decerebrate individual and is observed in those with severe mental delay, kernicterus, or CNS infections.

Obtain the *tonic neck reflex* by placing the child supine and turning the head to one side. The contralateral arm and leg flex and the ipsilateral arm and leg extend. The head is turned to the opposite side, and the position of the limbs reverses. In practice, the opposite flexion and extension may occur and the test may still be positive. This reflex is present at birth and normally lasts 3–5 months. If present after this time, brain damage should be suspected.

Inability to move the neck from side to side may accompany any of the previously named states and also occurs in congenital torticollis, the Klippel-Feil syndrome, and occasionally with cervical rib. Neurologic torticollis occurs in patients with lesions of the spinal accessory nerve, causing sternocleidomastoid and trapezius muscle paralysis, or it occurs without apparent cause. Eye lesions, especially when vision is unequal, or labyrinthitis, spasmus nutans, and brain tumors may be accompanied by torticollis. If the patient cannot maintain the head elevated (head drop), consider early poliomyelitis or other causes of muscle weakness.

Voluntary *tilting* of the neck may be seen in children with habit spasm, brain tumors, poor vision, or strabismus. Head-tilting from side to side may occur in children in whom the corpus callosum is absent. Head rolling and nodding may be due to habit spasm, mental retardation, eye or ear abnormalities, or chorea.

The Chest

Many disease states can be diagnosed by simply looking at the chest. Sometimes it is difficult to do more than observe a hyperactive or crying patient.

CHEST

The order of examination of the chest in a child depends on the attitude of the child; some physicians find it easier to listen to the chest first, before a young child starts to cry, and then to proceed with the other parts of the examination; others observe and palpate first and use the stethoscope later.

Inspection

Note the general *shape* and *circumference* of the chest. Obtain the chest circumference at the nipple line. It is normally the same as or slightly less than the head circumference for the first 2 years of life; it then exceeds the head circumference. In very sturdy children, the chest circumference is slightly greater than that of the head, even during the first 2 years. Marked disproportion between head and chest measurements requires comparison with standards for the child's age. Disproportions in children aged less than 2 years are usually caused by abnormal head growth rather than abnormal chest growth. When the measurements are compared with standards, however, the cause of abnormal growth can usually be determined. In children with respiratory disease, measure the chest in inspiration and expiration. The normal teenager can expand the chest at least 4–5 cm. Less expansion usually indicates intrathoracic pulmonary disease.

In premature infants, the rib cage is thin, and the chest may appear to collapse with every inspiration. In infancy, the chest is almost round, the anteroposterior diameter equaling the transverse diameter. As the child grows older, the chest normally expands in the transverse diameter. A round or emphysematous chest in a child after 6 years of age suggests a chronic pulmonary disease such as asthma. A funnel-shaped chest, pectus excavatum, characterized by sternal depression, may be a congenital anomaly or may indicate adenoid hypertrophy. A short, wide chest is noted especially in short children or in those with Morquio disease. *Pigeon breast*, pectus carinatum, in which the sternum protrudes, is noted as an isolated anomaly or in children with rickets or osteopetrosis. The *xiphisternum* may protrude and appear broken, but this condition is normal in young children and results only from a loose attachment between the xiphoid and the body of the sternum. As in adults, note is made of the rib numbers to orient the examiner. The second rib attaches at the angle of the sternum just below the clavicles.

When the patient is lying supine, swellings at the costochondral junction may be evident. These swellings or blunt knobbings form the *rachitic rosary*. Almost always a depression will be noted in the child in the region of the eighth to tenth ribs, and the bottom of the rib cage will appear to flare. The depression at the site of the diaphragm muscle leaving the chest wall is termed *Harrison's groove*. Although it occurs in rickets, this type of flaring is also common in many children with any pulmonary disorder, in children who were born prematurely, and in many normal young children who have no obvious pathologic disturbance. Edema of the chest wall occurs in children with superior vena cava obstruction, mediastinal compression syndrome, or mumps.

Note the *angle* made by the lower rib margin with the sternum. Ordinarily this angle is about 45 degrees. You may find a larger angle in children with lung disease and a smaller angle in those with malnutrition and deficiency states. Note *expansion* of the chest. Most of a child's normal respiratory activity is effected by abdominal motion until age 6 or 7 years, with very little intercostal motion. Later, thoracic motion becomes responsible for air exchange. If the interspaces show much motion with intercostal muscle retraction, lung disease or peritonitis is suggested. Note whether the motion of the interspaces is restricted to one side. Less motion occurs on the involved side, and increased motion occurs on the opposite side of the chest with pneumonia, hydrothorax or pneumothorax, obstructive foreign body, or atelectasis. Expiration is normally about two thirds the length of inspiration. Expiration is increased with obstruction in the larynx or trachea or in intrinsic pulmonary disease, such as asthma, pneumonitis, or cystic fibrosis.

These disease states and paralysis of the chest musculature also produce increased motion of the diaphragm. With normal respiration the chest expands, the sternal angle increases, and the diaphragm descends on inspiration; the reverse occurs with expiration. Paradoxical respiration is noted when the diaphragm appears to rise on inspiration and to descend on expiration. Paradoxical motion of the chest and diaphragm may be produced by any of the disease states mentioned, particularly pneumothorax. The side of the chest that is involved tends to collapse on inspiration and remains stationary or appears to expand on expiration. Paradoxical respiration is also noted in children with neuromuscular diseases such as phrenic nerve paralysis or chorea.

By observation, you can sometimes determine the difference between high obstruction and low obstruction. *Retraction* is chiefly suprasternal and severe in high obstruction, such as laryngeal lesions, but mainly infrasternal in low obstruction, such as infantile bronchiolitis. Retractions are usually less intense in lower obstruction. Diseases such as croup, congenital laryngeal stridor, stridor resulting from injury of the laryngeal nerves, diphtheria, and bronchiolitis; diseases of the abdomen such as peritonitis; and paralysis of the diaphragm also produce marked retraction above and below the sternum, with marked intercostal activity bilaterally.

Note *asymmetry*, Precordial bulging may indicate an interatrial septal defect, other causes of right or biventricular enlargement, pneumothorax, or a chronic localized chest disease. Lung tumors such as Ewing's sarcoma, as well as congenital absence of the chest muscles, may cause asymmetry; however, asymmetry is most commonly found secondary to scoliosis.

Chest Pain

Cardiac
- Mitral valve prolapse
- Pericarditis
- Coronary artery
  insufficiency
- Kawasaki disease
- Aortic stenosis
- Dysrrhythmias
- Pulmonary hypertension
- Dissecting aortic
  aneurysm
- Takayasu syndrome
- Myocarditis
- Embolism—thromboses
- Vasculitis
- Precordial catch
  syndrome

Noncardiac
- Trauma
- Muscle fatigue
- Asthma

Noncardiac (continued)
- Skin infections
- Collagen vascular diseases
- Pneumonia—bronchitis
- Pleuritis
- Pneumothorax
- Subcutaneous emphysema
- Tietze syndrome
- Adolescent breast
  development
- Cervical rib
- Slipping rib
- Scalenus-anticus syndrome
- Tumor
- Mediastinitis—
  pneumomediastinum
- Sickle cell disease, trait
- Leukemia, lymphoma
- Gastrointestinal, renal
  conditions
- Emotional
- Poisoning

Weakness or deficiency in the sternocleidomastoid or trapezoid muscles may result from injury to the spinal accessory nerve. Chest *pain* may be accompanied by tenderness and may be caused by extrathoracic or intrathoracic lesions or may be referred from other organs, such as the abdomen, spine, or neck. Pain over the lower ribs may follow trauma: pull the inferior rib margins anteriorly. The symptoms will be reproduced because of "slipping ribs."

Note the position of the scapulas for anomalies such as Sprengel deformity, winged scapula, and Klippel-Feil syndrome, which are described in the section on examination of the spine (Chapter 7).

BREASTS

Note breast development (Fig. 5-1). Breast development normally begins before pubic hair develops.

It may be difficult to determine whether a breast that appears large is hypertrophic or is truly developmentally enlarged. The hypertrophic breast usually has a flat nipple with a small areola, and the breast tissue feels soft. The developed breast usually has protrusion of the nipple, enlargement of the areola, and a firmness to the tissue underlying the areola. Redness, heat, and tenderness around the breast may indicate infection (mastitis). Ordinarily, do not palpate the neonatal breast, which is enlarged for about 1 or 2 months. Examine breasts during routine examinations after breast development begins, when breasts fail to develop, or when symptoms or problems occur.

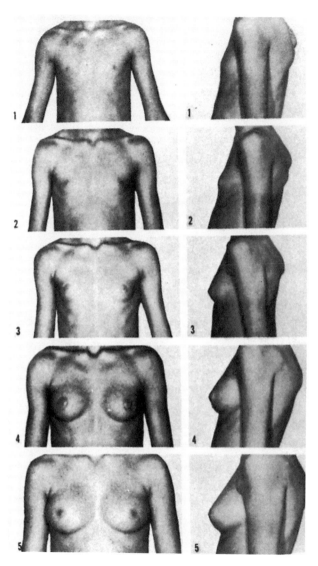

Figure 5-1. Breast development stages during adolescence. Stage 1, preadolescent (elevation of papillae). Stage 2, "bud" stage (elevation of breast and papillae with some increase in areolar diameter). Stage 3, enlargement (no separation of contours). Stage 4, projection (areolae and papillae from secondary mounds). Stage 5, mature (projection of only papillae and recession of areolae). (From Tahner JM. *Growth at adolescence.* Philadelphia: F.A. Davis, 1962.)

In girls, normal breast is less than 2 cm in diameter and development begins between the ages of 8 and 14 years. One breast usually begins to develop before the other and is frequently tender. With the patient in the supine position with the arm under the head, palpate in concentric circles inward from the axilla and clavicle to the areola for each side. Precocious breast development in girls is usually innocuous. Complete central isosexual precocity may be caused by central nervous system (CNS) defects or precocity from any cause. With precocious thelarche, linear growth rate is normal. With precocious puberty, linear growth rate is increased. Pseudoprecocious breast enlargement occurs in corpulent children and is merely the result of adipose tissue. In such "breasts," the tissue is softer than true breast tissue and cannot be distinguished from surrounding tissue.

Precocious Breast Development

Pseudoisosexual Precocity	Central Isosexual Precocity
Granulosa cell tumor	Septooptic dysplasia
Follicular cysts	Hydrocephalus
McCune-Albright syndrome	Cysts, brain trauma, brain tumors (e.g., hamartoma, neurofibroma, optic glioma, astrocytoma, irradiation, meningitis)
Oral contraceptives	
Adrenal feminizing tumors	
Hypothyroidism	
Hyperthyroidism	
Marijuana, opiates, amphetamines	
Stilbestrol ingestion	
Prescription drugs (e.g., digitalis, cimetidine, isoniazid, phenothiazines, antidepressants)	

Measure and diagram any lumps and repeat the examination 1 week after menses occur. A unilateral lump immediately under the areola is normal in developing tissue. In girls 8–10 years old and in boys 13–18 years old, subareolar masses immediately behind the areola that are firm, smooth, discoid, and 2–3 cm in diameter result from hyperplasia. These *masses* usually regress within 1 year. Small, round, hard *nodules* in the breasts of children, as in adults, may be caused by cysts or tumors. These masses are usually both nontender and irregular; they may feel attached to the skin or grow out of proportion to the remainder of the breast tissue. Swelling, tenderness, heat, and redness in nodules are signs of inflammation (e.g., cellulitis or abscess) and may follow ductal obstruction, injury, or infection in a cyst; these signs occur more commonly during periods of increased hormonal secretion. Tender nodules with ecchymosis indicate trauma.

Painless, circumscribed, firm masses may result from fat necrosis after an injury. These mobile masses may be fixed to the skin and must be distinguished from those immobile and not so sharply delineated masses that result from carcinoma. Small, mobile, circumscribed, tender masses that increase in tenderness during menses may represent periductal fibrosis, cystic ductal hyperplasia, adenosis, or lobular hyperplasia. Bilateral lumpy thickening occurs with fibrocystic disease. Nodules that are nontender, firm, freely movable, and sharply demarcated are usually fibroadenomas. The long curve of breast tissue extending into the axilla enlarges with hormonal surges.

True gynecomastia in boys usually results from unknown benign factors at puberty but may be caused by tumors of the breast, severe liver disease, drug usage and, very rarely, gonadal or adrenal lesions. Usually breast enlargement in boys is caused only by adipose tissue, but it may occur with gonadal dysgenesis, Klinefelter syndrome, or digitalis administration.

Breast development is absent in adolescent girls with pituitary failure, anorexia nervosa with onset before puberty, gonadal dysgenesis, adrenal hyperplasia, or severe malnutrition. Record the stage of development (Fig. 5-1).

Galactorrhea, a whitish discharge from the nipple, may be caused by pregnancy, hypothalamic or pituitary tumor such as prolactinoma or craniopharyngioma, or drug ingestion. A bloody discharge signals an intraductal papilloma, a purulent discharge suggests abscess, and a greenish-black discharge suggests duct ectasia.

LUNGS

Note the type and rate of breathing. A newborn, especially a premature baby, will normally have Cheyne-Stokes respirations, characterized by periods of deep and rapid respirations alternating with periods of slow, shallow respirations or no respiratory activity (*apnea*); this pattern should disappear by 4 weeks of life when breathing becomes regular. Various brain or metabolic lesions that depress the central respiratory center may cause Cheyne-Stokes respirations.

The *rate* of respiration varies from 30 to 80 breaths per minute (bpm) at birth, 20–60 bpm in infancy, 16–20 bpm at 6 years, and 14–20 bpm at puberty. Because young children tend to have an abnormally high respiratory rate when even slightly excited, estimation of true respiratory rate is best obtained when the infant or young child is asleep. Children with any type of respiratory disorder almost always have a rapid respiratory rate, *tachypnea*; a normal respiratory rate usually indicates lack of acute pulmonary disease. Children aged less than 3 years with upper airway obstruction rarely breathe at a rate faster than 50 bpm, whereas children with lower airway obstructive disease, such as bronchiolitis, frequently breathe at rates of 80–100 bpm. In young children, tachypnea may be an early sign of heart failure.

Children with generalized or localized infection, fever, poisoning, salicylism, acidosis, or shock also frequently have a rapid respiratory rate. A slow rate suggests central respiratory depression, especially that caused by increased intracranial pressure, sedatives or other drugs, alkalosis, or poisons. Slow, jerky respiratory movements or bursts of hyperpnea alternating with apnea (Biot breathing) may be noted in cases of CNS lesions involving the respiratory center, such as encephalitis.

Note the *depth* of respiration. Deep respirations are termed *hyperpnea*. Depth of respiration is an indication of the degree of anoxia present, the state of activity of the respiratory center, and the presence of acidosis or alkalosis.

In obstructive respiratory diseases, breathing is usually rapid and may be deep or shallow, depending on the degree and nature of the obstruction. In metabolic acidosis, breathing is deep; the respiratory rate is usually rapid but is depressed in alkalosis of long duration. Listening while holding the bell of the stethoscope over the mouth of a young child helps one estimate the rate and depth of respiration and frequently assists in diagnosing the degree of acidosis.

Establishing your own standards for depth of respiration is worthwhile. Examine a group of children aged 1,3,6,9, and 12 months and 1,2,3,4,5,6,8, and 10 years in both the normal standing posture and in the supine position. During normal respiration, air from the child's nose will be felt a measurable distance from the nose. Record this distance for each age. You can then use each figure, plus or minus 2 cm, as your norm. My measurements for these ages, when the patients are supine, are 4 and 6 cm for infants aged 1 and 3 months, respectively; 10 cm for 6,9, and 12 months; 12 and 15 cm for 1 and 2 years, respectively; 20 cm for 3 and 4 years; 22 cm for 5 and 6 years; and 25 cm for 8 and 10 years. You can determine increased depth of respiration by feeling the child's breath from a farther distance and decreased depth by feeling the child's breath closer to the child's nose.

Recognize *dyspnea*, or distress during breathing, by observing flaring of the nares and intercostal spaces, cyanosis, suprasternal and infrasternal retraction, and rapid respiratory rate. Try to note whether the distress is mainly inspiratory or expiratory; inspiratory distress occurs more frequently with high obstructions, and expiratory distress occurs with low obstructions. Distress in tracheal obstruction is both inspiratory and expiratory. Dyspnea may also occur with pulmonary infections, pain, fright, anemia, cardiovascular disorders, and hyperthyroidism.

Dyspnea is usually increased by exercise and forms the basis of the *exercise tolerance test*. If limitation of exercising ability is suspected, some type of graded measurement of this ability is desirable. Usually, children of various ages can be asked to run about or up and down stairs and are then compared with their peers for the development of dyspnea. Dyspnea that occurs too soon indicates any state that may cause anoxia or causes such as lack of habit of exercise, obesity, or emotional distress. Exercise of the arms causes more dyspnea than an equivalent amount of exercise of the lower extremities.

Cough may result from intrathoracic or extrathoracic causes. Expiratory paroxysmal cough followed by an inspiratory whoop in a child more than 6 months of age or followed by vomiting in a child less than 6 months of age is characteristic of pertussis, parapertussis, and respiratory infection even months after pertussis. A loose productive cough is noted in children with bronchitis, upper respiratory infection with postnatal drip, and cystic fibrosis with pulmonary involvement. A sharp, brassy, nonproductive, barking cough, which sounds like the bark of a seal, is heard in children with laryngeal diphtheria, foreign body obstruction, croup and, occasionally, tuberculosis. The child with

---

Cough

Intrathoracic Causes
- Reactive airway disease
- Allergies, asthma, fumes, drugs
- Cystic fibrosis
- Cardiac failure, emboli
- Foreign body in bronchi, atelectasis
- Masses (e.g., lymphoma, sarcoid, Wegener granulomatosis, tumors)

Infection
- Pneumonia, bronchitis, bronchiolitis
- Tracheitis
- Bacteria, viruses
- Viruses
- Protozoa, including *Pneumocystis carinii*
- Fungi (e.g., *Histoplasma, Aspergillus*)
- *Mycoplasma pneumoniae*
- Parasites (e.g., visceral larva migrans)
- *Chlamydia* (e.g., *C. trachomatis, C. psittaci*)
- *Rickettsia* (e.g., Q fever)
- Hydrocarbon ingestion

Anomalies
- Lobar emphysema, cyst, sequestration, vascular ring, tracheoesophageal fistula

Extrathoracic Causes
- Foreign body in ear, trachea, esophagus
- Smoking
- Tic, habit, emotion

Infection
- Upper respiratory, postnasal drip, pharyngitis, croup, laryngitis, sinusitis

Anomalies
- Cricopharyngeal incoordination, long uvula, laryngomalacia, immobile cilia

---

croup is usually 3 months to 5 years old, is in distress, and is in the supine position. A tight, nonproductive cough is heard with pneumonia. A staccato cough suggests chlamydial infection.

Cough is usually nonproductive in children, even those with tuberculosis or bronchiectasis, and *expectoration* is rare. Hemoptysis may indicate foreign body obstruction, tuberculosis, other pulmonary infections, trauma, tumors, heart disease, or bleeding from high in the respiratory tract. Children with chronic pulmonary disease may have purulent sputum. Children with measles, tracheitis, or laryngitis have a dry, irritative persistent cough.

You can usual elicit the *cough reflex* by examining the child's throat with a tongue blade or by placing your finger in the suprasternal notch and pressing, which causes the child to gag. The cough reflex may be depressed in children with mental retardation, debilitating disease, and paralysis of the respiratory musculature and in those who have received sedatives or cough depressants.

Palpation

Place the palm of your hand lightly but firmly on the patient's chest and feel with the palm and fingertips. Palpate the entire chest. Palpation confirms your observation of the chest wall, such as position of the scapulas, position or fracture of the clavicles, asymmetry of the chest, and the presence of rosary, Harrison groove, breast tissue, and axillary lymph nodes. Note any masses or areas of *tenderness*. A *thud* is occasionally palpated high on the chest as the patient breathes. This is a sign of foreign body in the trachea. Palpation of the heart is discussed later in this chapter.

Tactile fremitus is easily determined by palpating the chest wall in children who are crying, who can cooperate by speaking, or who can be asked their name. Fremitus, when obtainable, is usually felt over the entire chest as a tingling sensation. Decrease in fremitus suggests the presence of airway obstruction or may indicate pleural effusion. When the patient does not make vocal sounds, fremitus is normally absent, but it is frequently felt in children who have been crying and signifies a partial movable obstruction to the passage of air. Tactile fremitus is especially valuable in distinguishing the presence of mucus high in the respiratory tract, where fremitus is very coarse, from lower respiratory tract infection, where it is absent. Fremitus is a poor sign for distinguishing pneumonia, atelectasis, or space-occupying lesions in a child.

Palpate the rib interspaces for retraction and *paralysis* of the intercostal muscles. Intercostal retraction is caused by increased work of breathing. Intercostal bulging during expiration indicates expiratory obstruction.

Decreased motion of the interspaces may indicate paralysis of the intercostal muscles, decreased respiratory activity, or, if unilateral, any of the causes of decreased respiration of one side of the chest. Subcostal retraction of the diaphragm with hyperinflation of the chest suggests air trapping. *Pulsation* of the rib vessels from coarctation of the aorta usually occurs in the teen years. Pericardial or pleural friction rubs can occasionally be palpated and feel like fine vibrations. A crackling sensation under your fingers may result from subcutaneous emphysema or a bone fracture.

The axillary lymph nodes are palpated best by bringing the palm of your hand flat into the axilla with the patient's arm hanging freely at the side. A slight rubbing motion will indicate the size of the glands. Normally, several glands as large as 3 mm in diameter will be felt in all children. Abnormalities of these nodes are described in the section on lymph nodes (Chapter 3).

Percussion

Use direct and indirect methods in percussion of the chest. In the direct method (Fig. 5-2) the chest wall is tapped lightly with either the index or the middle finger. Every centimeter of the chest is percussed quickly. This method is rapid, gentle, and informative but requires considerable practice.

For the indirect method of percussion, place a finger of one hand firmly on the patient's chest wall; use the index or middle finger of the other hand as the percussing hammer and cover the same areas. The bases for good indirect percussion are (a) the nonpercussing finger must be pressed *firmly* against the chest wall; (b) no other fingers should touch the chest wall; (c) the patient should be sitting, standing, or lying flat on the back or abdomen; and (d) the

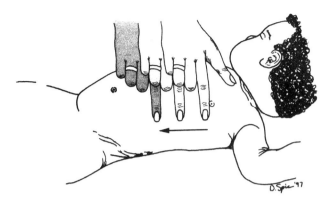

Figure 5-2. Direct percussion.

percussing finger should move like a piano hammer, with a very loose hinge-joint action at the wrist. Because the chest wall is thinner and the muscles are smaller, the chest is more resonant in children than in adults. Therefore, accurate information is much more easily attained by examining the chest of a child. If you percuss too vigorously, however, vibrations over a large area may obscure localized areas of dullness.

Posteriorly, percuss from the shoulders down to dullness at the level of the eighth to tenth ribs, where the diaphragm causes a change in the note. It is important that the patient's head be in the midline position facing directly forward during this part of the examination. If the neck is twisted, aeration is not equal, and spurious dullness may be detected. The top of the diaphragm is usually located at about the level of the apex of the costovertebral angle. Anteriorly, tap from just below the clavicle to the level of dullness. Percuss the sides of the chest from the axillae downward. Then, starting at the lower margin of the lung fields posteriorly and the upper abdomen anteriorly, determine the lower margins and the mobility of the diaphragm. It is generally useful to begin percussing in the areas where resonance is expected and continue to where dullness is expected. This is especially important over the area of the heart.

You will find a decreased percussion note, or *dullness*, over the scapulas, diaphragm, liver, and heart. Demarcate these areas. Normally the top of the liver is percussed anteriorly at about the level of the sixth rib from the midaxillary line to the sternum. The lower edge of the lung or the top of the diaphragm is usually percussed to the level of the eighth to tenth ribs posteriorly on both sides. Anteriorly, the diaphragm usually cannot be percussed below the level of the liver on the right. Occasionally, because a distended stomach will cause hyperresonance on the left, you may have difficulty delineating the level of the diaphragm. Fortunately, most children have an indentation of the ribs at the attachment of the diaphragm to help indicate where dullness is expected. Usually the diaphragm is also percussed anteriorly at the level of the eighth to the tenth rib. In all these areas, the diaphragm will usually move, as determined by changing dullness, one to two rib spaces between inspiration and expiration. In a child aged less than 2 years, this motion is very difficult to determine by percussion.

These normal areas of percussion dullness may be altered as follows: Liver dullness may be determined at a level higher than the sixth rib in conditions causing liver enlargement; elevation of the liver, as in abdominal distention; or in atelectasis of the lobes of the right lung. The liver will be percussed at the level of the sixth rib on the left in dextrocardia with levorotation of the liver or with situs inversus. The diaphragm will be higher than normal in conditions causing collapse of the lungs or distention of the abdomen and will be lower than normal in conditions causing emphysema of the lungs with masses or space occupying lesions in the chest.

The mediastinum in children is usually percussed as the area of cardiac dullness. Rarely, a broadened area of dullness above or at the level of the heart may be caused by the thymus. Although this is without significance, note any broadening of the mediastinum, since it may indicate presence of other masses. Heart dullness will be altered by conditions causing a shift of the heart or mediastinum. Localized areas of decreased resonance, dullness, or flatness may be found.

Areas of Dullness

Lung	Pleura
Consolidation	Effusion
Collapse (atelectasis)	Emphysema
Tumor	
Edema	

Left effusion more likely results from pancreatic disease. Right effusion is more likely caused by heart failure or ovarian disease. Dullness below the angle of the left scapula may occur with pericardial effusion (Ewart or Pin sign).

Hyperresonance of the chest is caused by an increase in the amount of air in the chest. It is most common in children with emphysema and is usually accompanied by a lowered diaphragm. Localized hyperresonance may also indicate the presence of free air in the chest (such as pneumothorax) or the presence of loculated air (such as lung cyst or abscess, obstructive foreign body, or diaphragmatic hernia). Increase in resonance over the area of the liver may indicate a ruptured abdominal viscus.

Auscultation

The inside of the stethoscope should be clean and the tubing intact, well fitting, and about 45 cm long. Warm the stethoscope before use and press it firmly against the chest wall, or sounds that are artifacts will be heard. A tight fit of the stethoscope with the chest is usually accomplished more easily if the bell is placed in the interspaces rather than over the ribs. If the stethoscope is not firmly placed on the chest, nothing will be heard. Auscultate the entire chest, including the axillary areas. Children's fingers must sometimes be restrained from touching the tubing during this part of the examination because touching the tubing also makes extraneous sounds. Listen for breath sounds, rales, rhonchi, and extraneous sounds. Especially during auscultation, the child should be completely supine or totally erect, since even a slight turning of the head may decrease the breath sounds and suggest pathologic states. Because of the small size of the child's chest and the need to localize pathologic findings and to avoid the scratch sounds made by chest hair, the small bell stethoscope is most satisfactory for auscultation in children.

Breath sounds may seem much louder in children than in adults because of the thinness of the chest wall. Inspiration is three times as long as expiration with vesicular sounds, twice as long with bronchovesicular; expiration is slightly longer with bronchial sounds, and inspiration and expiration are about equal with sounds originating from the trachea. Because breath sounds in a child are almost all bronchovesicular or even bronchial, sound quality offers little help in diagnosis. Decreased breath sounds indicate decreased air flow and are noted especially in children with bronchopneumonia, atelectasis, pleural effusion, pneumothorax, and empyema. Increased breath sounds are sometimes heard with resolving pneumonia. Bronchial breath sounds may be heard over areas of consolidation in the older child. Auscultate the area over the mediastinum in the midline both anteriorly and posteriorly. Normally you will hear no breath sounds over the sternum or vertebrae. Increased breath sounds will be heard in these areas in the presence of consolidation.

Inspiratory *rales* are usually heard as fine crackles. They may be heard throughout the chest in infants and children with bronchiolitis, bronchopneumonia, pulmonary edema, or atelectasis. Rales heard exclusively in the upper part of the chest are more commonly associated with cystic fibrosis. Rales in the lower chest are more common in children with heart failure. Rales heard only late in inspiration are more indicative of interstitial lung disease such as fibrosing alveolitis.

The presence of fine rales may be clarified in children, as in adults, by having the patient cough at the end of expiration. Demonstrate exactly the procedure you expect the child to perform. Even young children can sometimes be induced to cough in this manner. Rales that disappear after coughing usually have no significance.

Frequently you will hear inspiratory rales only at the very end of inspiration or only after deep inspiration. Because a crying child inspires deeply before each cry, auscultation may be quite informative during crying. Instruct slightly older children to blow against your hand, or tell them to blow out the otoscope light or to blow on a pinwheel; they will usually inspire deeply before blowing. Instruct still older children to breath deeply through the mouth, especially if you demonstrate this type of breathing.

Expiratory rales or crackles are prominent in bronchiolitis, cystic fibrosis, asthma, and foreign body aspiration. Rales are mainly expiratory with intrathoracic obstruction to air flow, inspiratory with extrathoracic obstruction, or both with severe obstruction either in or outside the chest.

Pleural *friction rub* is a coarse grating sound heard through the stethoscope with each respiration, as though it were close to your ear, and occurs occasionally with pneumonia, lung abscess, tuberculosis, or empyema. A loud slap may be heard high on the chest in a child with a tracheal foreign body obstruction. A crunching sound near the heart and synchronous with the heart-beat occurs with left pneumothorax (Hamman sign) or with pneumomediastinum.

Rhonchi caused by crying or upper respiratory infection may be inspiratory or expiratory and are coarse sounds. You can best distinguish them from rales by tactile fremitus or by holding the bell stethoscope over the mouth and comparing the sounds from the mouth with those over the chest. If similar, the sounds are originating high in the respiratory tract near the larynx. Any sound, especially if musical, that sounds the same over different areas of the chest almost invariably arises from the larynx or high in the trachea.

Wheezes are produced by airflow through compromised larger airways and usually sound more musical or sonorous than rales or rhonchi. Wheezes are heard more commonly in expiration than in inspiration and usually indicate partial obstruction during the expiratory phase, as occurs in children with bronchospasm. Inspiratory wheezes usually are heard in children with high obstruction, such as laryngeal edema or a foreign body; expiratory wheezes are usually heard in children with low obstruction, such as asthma or bronchiolitis. High-pitched wheezes are associated with severe asthma. Absence of wheezes in an asthmatic patient is a sign of a very severe disease. Crunching sounds heard during different phases of respiration may be caused by subcutaneous emphysema.

Vocal resonance can be obtained in children if they are induced to count, speak, or tell their names repeatedly. Increased resonance may indicate consolidation, and decreased resonance may indicate obstruction to flow of air.

Peristalsis is frequently heard over the left lower chest anteriorly because of the proximity of the bowel. However, peristalsis in the chest, particularly on the left side, may be a cardinal sign of diaphragmatic hernia. Murmur or bruits over the posterior lungs may be vascular or may occur with a sequestered lobe of the lung.

HEART

> *Soft is the heart of a child*
> *Do not harden it.*
>
> *Glenconner*

Certain basic information must be part of every examination of the heart: *rate, rhythm, size, shape, quality* of sounds, *murmurs* and *thrills, femoral pulses*, and *blood pressure*. In the routine examination of the heart, it is advantageous to evaluate the patient in several different positions if possible.

Pulse

Palpate the radial, femoral, and carotid pulses in young children and the tibial pulse in older children. Absent femoral pulse indicates coarctation of the aorta; absence of the other pulses occurs with Takayusu syndrome or later stages of diabetes.

The normal pulse rate varies from 70 to 170 beats per minute (beats/min) at birth to 120–140 beats/min soon after birth. Rates of 80–140 beats/min at 1 year, 80–130 beats/min at 2 years, 80–120 at 3 years and 70–115 after 3 years are within normal limits. By age 10 years, the normal rate decreases to 90 beats/min and in adolescence to 60–100 beats/min. Boys generally have slower rates than girls. After age 2 years, the pulse rate during sleep is usually 20 beats/min less than during wakening. Almost always, the pulse rate during sleep as well as during waking hours is elevated in active rheumatic fever, any other active infection, or thyrotoxicosis.

Tachycardia

Excitement	Hyperthyroid
Exercise	Digitalis toxicity
Fever	Heart disease
Neuroblastoma	Pheochromocytoma
Systemic diseases	Toxins

In rheumatic fever, in contrast to other infections, the increased rate is usually out of proportion to the increase in temperature. The pulse rate is usually increased by 10–15 bpm for each centigrade degree of fever. In children with upper airway obstruction, pulse rates of 140–160 beats/min are common; in those with lower airway obstruction, rates may be 180–200 beats/min or more.

Supraventricular *tachycardia* with rates as high as 200–300 beats/min is sometimes noted in children with congenital heart or acquired myocardial diseases or with toxic states. An idiopathic auricular tachycardia may be a cause of sudden death in infancy. *Pulsus alternans*, in which one beat is strong and the next weak, is a sign of severe heart strain. A slow rate (*bradycardia*), less than 100 beats/min in infants and less than 60 beats/min in older children, frequently means some degree of heart block. In infancy, it is usually associated with a septal defect, digitalis poisoning, severe sepsis and, occasionally, hypothyroidism. In young teenagers, sinus bradycardia, especially with sinus arrhythmia, is common. Rare causes of slow pulse include carotid sinus hypersensitivity, hypercalcemia, hyperkalemia, increased intracranial pressure and, occasionally, acute myocarditis. The slow pulse rate sometimes noted in children with hypertension in acute nephritis may be related to an associated increased intracranial pressure. Slow rates may be noted in well-trained athletes.

Water-hammer, or Corrigan pulse, is felt as an especially forceful beat resulting from a very wide pulse pressure. It is noted best over either the radial or femoral arteries. Capillary pulsations, or Quincke pulse, which is noted most easily after you press lightly on the tip of the nail, also result from increased pulse pressure. A method sometimes used for eliciting capillary pulsations is rubbing of the skin of the child's forehead vigorously for a minute until generalized erythema appears. Observation reveals intermittent reddening and blanching in children with increased capillary pressures. Both these pulse types are found especially in older children with patent ductus arteriosus, aortic regurgitation, or peripheral arteriovenous fistula.

Thready pulse is a rapid, weak pulse that seems to appear and disappear. It is usually a sign of circulatory failure, shock, or heart failure. A dicrotic pulse feels as though it has a notch in it. You may find it in children with sepsis. The normal pulse has this notch, but it cannot usually be palpated. *Pulsus paradoxus* is a marked change in pulse amplitude with respiration. Take the blood pressure several times rapidly in different parts of the respiratory cycle. Alternatively, lower pressure in the cuff 1 mm/sec. Listen for the first faint sporadic sounds and the point at which all sounds are repetitive and crisp. Normally blood pressure does not increase more than 10 mm Hg in expiration. Children with well-developed thoracic respiration may exhibit greater differences. An increase of more than 10 mm Hg may be a sign of cardiac tamponade caused by pericardial effusion or constrictive pericarditis. A pulse pressure between two beats more than 20 mm Hg is a grave sign in a child with asthma, and with cystic fibrosis such an increase reflects severity of disease process. Reverse pulsus paradoxus, an increase in blood pressure with inspiration, is caused by an increase in left ventricular stroke output as in hypertrophic subaortic stenosis or during positive pressure breathing.

Almost all children, especially young adolescents, normally have sinus arrhythmia. Occasional runs of premature beats or of extrasystoles are common in childhood and may have no clinical significance. Regular rhythm in childhood is not rare but, if present, may indicate active carditis. You will rarely see auricular fibrillation in childhood because its chief cause—rheumatic heart disease—develops in older children or adults after childhood rheumatic fever. Arrhythmias, particularly ventricular, may cause syncope and may occur in patients with long QT intervals. Premature contractions that disappear after exercise are benign.

Inspection

In the routine examination of the heart, inspect the chest for precordial bulging, a sign of right-sided enlargement, and the visible cardiac *impulse* and its localization and diffuseness. Frequently the cardiac impulse is noted in normal children or in children who are hyperactive, thin, or excited. It is not visible in many normal children. If the impulse appears diffuse, it may be normal. The position of the impulse sometimes provides a rough idea of the heart size because it may correspond to the location of the apex of the heart.

Other observations made as part of the routine examination of the heart include the appearance of respiratory distress, cyanosis, edema, clubbing of the fingers, capillary pulsations, prominence of veins, and abnormal pulsations of neck and epigastric veins. The presence or absence of femoral pulses and the blood pressure also help in determining the status of the heart.

The size of the heart is the best indicator of the presence of heart disease. Heart size can be estimated by physical examination alone with careful inspection, palpation, and percussion.

Palpation

Palpation is useful in detecting the apex impulse (point of maximal impulse, PMI) of the heart. Although the PMI is an important physical sign in children and even in adolescents, it does not accurately reflect heart size. A more reliable guide is the apex beat. This is the position farthest toward the axilla and toward the lower rib margin which can be easily palpated. The apex beat is normally at the fifth interspace in the midclavicular line after age 7 years. Before this age, the apex beat is normally felt in the fourth interspace just to the left of the midclavicular line. The apex is usually at a lower interspace and more lateral in children with cardiac enlargement; pericardial effusion and various lung, spine, and chest wall diseases may also displace the apex.

The apex impulse may be difficult to feel in children aged less than 2 years or in children with pericardial effusion, heart failure, or emphysema. A forceful apex beat is felt in children after exercise or excitement or in those with thin chest walls, impending heart failure, fever, or hyperthyroidism.

Occasionally you can distinguish right ventricular hypertrophy from left ventricular hypertrophy by palpation. Place your palm over the child's sternum with your fingertips at the apex. Pulsation below and to the left of the apex indicates left ventricular enlargement; with right ventricular hypertrophy, you usually feel the impulse as a sharp tap or as a heave more medially. A sustained lift in the xiphoid region indicates right ventricular overwork. A slow heave suggests increased pressure work; a sharper hyperdynamic tap suggests increased volume work.

Usually the first (systolic) sound, occasionally the second (diastolic) sound and, in a failing heart, a third sound (gallop rhythm) may be palpated. Occasionally the child will complain of tenderness when the heart area is palpated. This does not indicate that heart disease is present or absent.

Vibratory thrills and pericardial friction rubs may also be palpated. They are felt as fine or coarse vibrations, either continuously or during some part of the cardiac cycle. Record position of cardiac thrills and their timing in the cardiac cycle. Obtain timing by simultaneously feeling either the apex impulse or the carotid pulse. Thrills at the apex are more easily felt with the child lying on their left side; basal thrills are more easily felt with the child sitting up.

A high-frequency thrill along the left sternal border suggests ventricular septal defect, a low-frequency midsystolic thrill in the second left interspace indicates pulmonic stenosis; a midsystolic thrill in the second right interspace suggests aortic stenosis, and a continuous thrill indicates patent ductus arteriosus. Feel also with one finger in the suprasternal notch. If the notch is very pulsatile, suspect patent ductus arteriosus (PDA) or aortic insufficiency. A diastolic thrill at the apex is usually caused by mitral stenosis.

Percussion

Percussion of the heart, like percussion of the lungs, may be performed by either the direct or indirect method. Scratch-percussion is an excellent way of determining cardiac borders. With the stethoscope over the heart, make longitudinal parallel scratches with a finger beginning in the axillary line and move toward the heart at about 1-cm intervals. As soon as the scratches are over the heart, you will detect a change in intensity of the scratch sound through the stethoscope (Fig. 5-3).

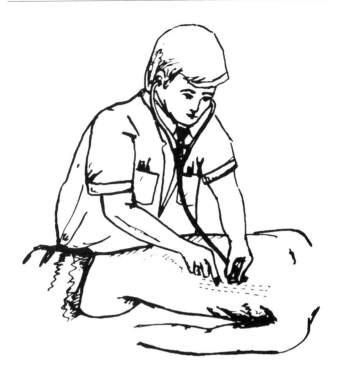

Figure 5-3. Scratch percussion. The stethoscope is near the sternum; parallel scratches are made down the left side of the chest.

In estimating heart size and shape, you may find a combined method of percussion and auscultation even more satisfactory. Place the stethoscope firmly on the child's chest just to the right of the sternum. Tap the chest wall lightly with your index finger, beginning in the axillary line and proceeding medially. As soon as your finger is tapping over the heart, you will note a sharp increase in sound.

The heart is usually percussed easily as a triangular area with one side of the triangle extending along the right sternal border from the second to the fifth rib, one side extending from the right sternal to the left midclavicular line along the fifth rib, and the third side extending from the right sternal border at the second rib to the left midclavicular line at the fifth rib. Usually, the heart of the infant is more horizontal, and the apex of the left border dullness (LBD) is to the left of the nipple line.

The area of heart dullness may be altered in a child with a normal or abnormal heart size. In right or left ventricular hypertrophy, you may percuss the heart at a lower interspace or more laterally. Percussion dullness to the right of the sternum in the third or fourth interspace usually indicates right-sided heart enlargement or dextrocardia. Right-sided enlargement produces precordial bulging.

Heart Strain or Enlargement

Right	Left
Pulmonic stenosis	Coarctation of aorta
Intraatrial septal defect	Tricuspid atresia
Congenital heart lesion	Endocardial fibroelastosis
Mitral stenosis	Glycogen storage disease
	Aberrant coronary artery
	Aberrant pulmonary vein
	Hypertension

Dullness to the left of the midclavicular line suggests left ventricular enlargement. In children with emphysema or space-occupying lesions in the chest, the heart is pushed away from the lesion, whereas in children with atelectasis, the heart is pulled toward the side of the lesion. The heart normally moves a little as the patient is turned from side to side. If motion does not occur when the patient is turned, pulmonary masses or adhesions may be present. This physical finding is rare in childhood, however. The heart may be percussed far to the left in the second and third interspace when the child is recumbent, and it may be in the normal position when the child sits. This change in position may indicate the presence of pericardial effusion.

Small hearts, characteristic of patients with Addison disease or constrictive pericarditis, are rare in childhood. An enlarged heart is characteristic of almost all types of heart disease: congenital heart disease with heart strain, anemia, myocarditis, or rheumatic fever. Less common causes of enlarged heart include endocardial fibroelastosis, pericardial effusion, patent ductus arteriosus, hypertension in nephritis, tumors, glycogen storage disease, or peripheral arteriovenous shunt. Patent ductus arteriosus may be present with a normal-sized heart.

Auscultation

Auscultate as you do when auscultating the lungs. Listen with the child in the sitting and supine positions. Use both the bell and the diaphragm over the entire precordium, paying special reference to the valve areas as in adults: The areas shown in Fig. 5-4 are the listening posts of the valve areas and not the true or anatomic valve areas. These areas regularly include the mitral valve at the apex, the pulmonary valve at the second interspace to the left of the sternum, the aortic valve at the second interspace to the right of the sternum (and at the third left interspace for diastolic murmurs), and the tricuspid valve in the fourth interspace over the sternum. In addition to auscultating in these areas, in children auscultate just to the right of the apex and several centimeters to the left of the sternum in the third interspace (frequent sites of innocent murmurs), along the sternal border (site of murmurs of septal defects), the second and third interspaces several centimeters to the left of the sternum (sites of murmurs of patent ductus arteriosus and coarctation of the aorta), above the clavicles (sites of venous hums and transmitted murmurs), and in the axillae, along the left midaxillary line, and below the scapulae (sites of transmitted murmurs). In children, auscultation will usually yield a better measurement of the cardiac rate than will palpation at the wrist.

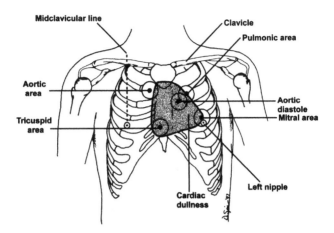

Figure 5-4.   Listening areas of the heart.

Evaluate the quality of the sounds. The first sound is best heard with the bell and the second is best heard with the diaphragm. In newborns, sounds should be sharp and clear. Distant sounds may indicate pericardial fluid, atelectasis, or another pulmonary disease. Sounds of poor quality, those that do not sound clear but are slurred or "mushy," are almost always characteristic of severe heart disease or myocarditis, usually with heart failure. In newborns, both sounds are of approximate equal intensity. Later, the apical first sound is louder than the second, and the pulmonic second sound is louder than the first in childhood.

A loud, snapping apical first sound is heard with mitral stenosis, left-to-right shunt, or conditions with high cardiac output; a decreased apical first sound is heard in early myocarditis.

In pulmonic stenosis, pulmonic atresia, or truncus, the pulmonic second sound usually is decreased or absent. The pulmonic second sound is normally louder than the aortic second sound during childhood and is very loud in pulmonary hypertension. You may hear the pulmonic second sound better in the third than in the second left interspace in children. The aortic second sound is usually diminished in intensity with aortic stenosis and acute myocarditis. In aortic insufficiency, the aortic second sound is often increased, but it may be decreased or absent. The aortic second sound is increased in children with hypertension of any cause. The tricuspid first sound may be obliterated with tricuspid regurgitation, a rare congenital anomaly.

The first sound, S_1, results from mitral and tricuspid (atrioventricular) valve closure. When the first sound is *split*, the first component is caused by mitral closure. The second sound, S_2, results from aortic and pulmonic valve closure, the aortic valve closing slightly before the pulmonic. Splitting of the second sound is heard best in the pulmonic area and is common in normal children. Deep inspiration delays pulmonic valve closure

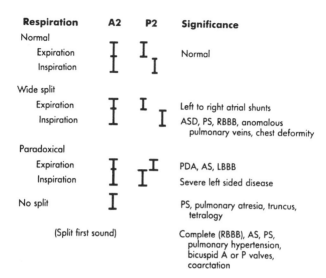

Respiration	A2	P2	Significance
Normal			
Expiration			Normal
Inspiration			
Wide split			
Expiration			Left to right atrial shunts
Inspiration			ASD, PS, RBBB, anomalous pulmonary veins, chest deformity
Paradoxical			
Expiration			PDA, AS, LBBB
Inspiration			Severe left sided disease
No split			PS, pulmonary atresia, truncus, tetralogy
(Split first sound)			Complete (RBBB), AS, PS, pulmonary hypertension, bicuspid A or P valves, coarctation

Figure 5-5. Second heart sounds splitting: A, aortic valve; P, pulmonic valve; AS, aortic stenosis; ASD, atrial septal defect; LBBB, left bundle branch block; PDA, patent ductus arteriosus; PS, pulmonic stenosis; RBBB, right bundle branch block.

and increases the splitting of the second sound (Fig. 5-5). Learn to appreciate splitting by first listening at the apex when aortic valve closure is simultaneous with mitral valve opening. Then move the stethoscope up, interspace by interspace, to the pulmonic area where the pulmonic valve closure is most distinct; two sounds will be heard. A third heart sound, S_3, is caused by vibration of the left ventricle wall, is present in about one third of children before puberty, and occurs between the second and first heart sound early in diastole. It is best heard at the apex, with a longer interval between the second and third sounds (usually with differing intensities and qualities), and occurs in mitral insufficiency or atrial septal defect. Later in diastole, just before the first sound, a fourth sound, S_4, may be audible and indicates decreased ventricular compliance, as in fibrosis or hypertrophy.

Either the first or second sound may be split in any valvular area without being a cause of concern. Four criteria are useful in distinguishing split sounds from a third heart sound: intensity, quality, position heard, and distance between sounds. Split second sounds are of equal quality and intensity, are heard most frequently at the base of the heart, and occur with a very short interval between the sounds.

Split second sounds at the base of the heart are common in children with conditions causing left-to-right shunts such as atrial septal defect, mild pulmonic stenosis, or right bundle branch block (Fig. 5-5). Splitting at the base is absent in children with pulmonic stenosis, tetralogy of Fallot, pulmonic atresia, or truncus. The wide splitting characteristically heard in children with atrial septal defects remains constant during inspiration

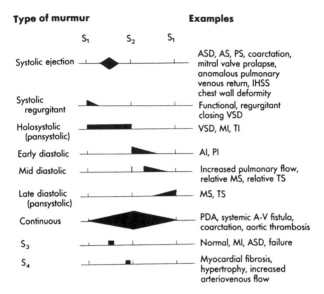

Figure 5-6. Types of murmurs and examples. AI, aortic insufficiency; AS, aortic stenosis; ASD, atrial septal defect; A-V, arteriovenous; IHSS, idiopathic hypertrophic subaortic stenosis; MI, mitral insufficiency; MS, mitral stenosis; PDA, patent ductus arteriosus; PI, pulmonic insufficiency; PS, pulmonic stenosis; TI, tricuspid insufficiency; TS, tricuspid stenosis; VSD, ventricular septal defect.

and expiration. Paradoxical splitting, a wider split in expiration than inspiration, occurs with patent ductus, aortic stenosis, complete left bundle branch block, or other severe left-sided lesions.

Clicks are high-pitched sounds you may hear when valves open. They may indicate aortic, pulmonic, or mitral valve stenosis or mitral valve prolapse. Low-pitched snaps in the mitral area occur in mitral stenosis.

Occasionally it is difficult to distinguish the third heart sound from a *gallop* rhythm, which indicates a failing heart. You may feel the three beats of the gallop on palpation; you can never feel the third heart sound as an impulse. Differentiation between the third sound and gallop rhythm is usually based on the presence of other evidence of heart disease, when gallop rhythm would be more likely to be heard than a third heart sound. *Tic-tac* rhythm, or embryocardia, exists if both sounds are almost alike in quality and intensity and are equidistant from each other. Although normal in younger children, this rhythm in older children may indicate a failing heart.

A difficult diagnostic feature in physical examination of children is determination of the significance of *murmurs*. Many children have murmurs without heart disease, and occasionally newborns or others have severe heart disease with no murmurs. Systolic murmurs are those that occur at or after the first and before the second sound; diastolic murmurs occur at or after the second and before the first sound. Murmurs heard in systole are early systolic (regurgitant), midsystolic, or pansystolic (holosystolic). Holosystolic murmurs are caused by blood flow from a chamber with higher pressure to a chamber with lower pressure. Diastolic murmurs may be early (protodiastolic) or middiastolic or may occur late in diastole (presystolic) (Fig. 5-6).

Describe quality of murmurs as soft, harsh, blowing, or whistling. Grade the intensity of murmurs. According to one system of grading, a grade-1 murmur is the softest possible murmur heard. It is not heard in all positions, especially not when the patient sits up or after exercise. A grade-2 murmur is the weakest murmur heard in all positions or after exercise. A grade-3 murmur is loud but is not accompanied by a thrill. A grade-4 murmur is loud but has a thrill. A grade-5 murmur is heard with the stethoscope barely on the chest. A grade-6 murmur can be heard with the stethoscope not touching the chest.

The intensity of murmurs alone does not indicate whether the murmur is significant of heart disease, although murmurs of grade 3 or louder usually do indicate heart disease. Following the intensity of a murmur over a period of hours, days, or weeks is helpful in determining the course of the heart disease. This is especially true in cases of rheumatic fever and bacterial endocarditis, in which the quality of the murmurs may change rapidly.

Murmurs may "rumble" for a short distance around the site of their maximal intensity but "radiate" or are "transmitted" if they are heard with distinct intensity some distance away from that site. Innocent murmurs usually do not radiate, and they may change in character with phase of respiration or change in position—being louder when the patient is supine than when the patient is in the sitting position. Innocent murmurs may appear or disappear during fever, exercise, excitement, or anemia. Any diastolic murmur or a murmur that is transmitted or radiates indicates heart disease.

Cardiopulmonary murmurs are soft, high-pitched sounds caused by the apposition of the heart and lungs, occur always in the same phase of respiration, can be obliterated by changing position, and usually have no pathologic significance but may indicate the presence of pleural adhesions. Murmurs indicating pleural adhesions are usually short, high-pitched and squeaking, are louder during inspiration, and project to the left sternal border. Murmurs originating from the left side of the heart are best heard in expiration.

Short-blowing, early systolic or midsystolic murmurs of low pitch heard best in the pulmonary area (usually in early adolescence), pulmonary flow murmurs, or vibratory murmurs that sound like musical buzzing over the precordium (in younger children) are usually innocent. If these murmurs radiate, they usually radiate downward; if murmurs of mitral insufficiency (MI) radiate, they usually radiate laterally. In addition, the murmur of MI is continuous during systole and is at or lateral to the apex; the innocent murmur, which is short, is usually medial to the apex in the general area where the murmurs of septal defects are heard.

A midsystolic, crescendo/decrescendo, loud, harsh murmur, ("diamond-shaped," "ejection") over the pulmonic area is characteristic of pulmonic stenosis (PS) and is also heard with atrial septal defects (ASD) or anomalous pulmonary venous return. This murmur is usually louder, harsher, and longer than the innocent murmur resulting from pulmonary flow. Peripheral pulmonic stenosis is accompanied by a soft systolic murmur over one or both lung fields but not over the heart. Pulmonic stenosis murmur may also be accompanied by a thrill and a systolic ejection click. A similar murmur in the second interspace just to the right of the sternum is characteristic of aortic stenosis (AS) or subaortic stenosis. This murmur radiates to the back. Atrial septal defect (ASD) is distinguished by fixed splitting of the second sound, increased intensity of the second component to the second sound at the upper left sternal edge and at the apex, and an early diastolic rumble from tricuspid flow audible at the midleft sternal border. Murmurs of aortic outflow radiate to the neck and may cause a carotid thrill. An aortic systolic murmur, which varies in intensity, may indicate idiopathic hypertrophic subaortic stenosis (IHSS), a dominantly inherited trait. It increases on standing and may be associated with mitral systolic murmur. A mid- or late-blowing systolic murmur, frequently beginning with multiple systolic clicks, is characteristic of mitral valve prolapse. Murmurs of mitral valve prolapse may be "honking" or "whooping."

The murmurs of septal defects and PS may be heard alone as isolated congenital anomalies or in combination, as in tetralogy of Fallot. The pulmonic systolic murmur with a loud tricuspid valve closure, split second sound, and prominent precordial activity may result from anterior displacement of a normal heart as in the straight back syndrome.

Holosystolic murmurs are common with mitral or tricuspid valve incompetence (MI, TI) and septal defects. In these, the first sound is not heard. Detection of this murmur very early in systole distinguishes it from innocent murmur. Marked changes in murmurs with respiration are usually caused by left heart lesions (e.g., ventricular septal defect or mitral regurgitation).

Diastolic murmurs that begin loud and then diminish in intensity are decrescendo [e.g., the murmur of aortic or pulmonic insufficiency (AI, PI)]. At the apex of the heart, murmurs starting softly and increasing in intensity are crescendo murmurs, like the murmurs of mitral stenosis (MS) or tricuspid stenosis (TS) resulting from valvular disease or increased flow secondary to a left-to-right shunt. Presystolic murmurs are usually associated with active atrial contraction and with mitral or tricuspid valve.

A continuous murmur in the second or third interspace to the left of the sternum that is widely transmitted is characteristic of PDA. A hum or high-pitched murmur anywhere along the course of the aorta may be a result of coarctation of the aorta or, rarely, a thrombosis of the aorta. A continuous murmur in the right or left parasternal areas may indicate a coronary or other arteriovenous fistula.

Rheumatic carditis is a type of acquired heart disease. A harsh, systolic, high-pitched or soft blow, sometimes obliterating the first sound and lasting through systole up to the second sound or beginning in late systole with crescendo to the second sound at or just to the right of the apex, may be the first sign of carditis and is usually caused by MI. This murmur is usually transmitted to the axilla or back. Later, an early diastolic or mid-diastolic crescendo blow in the same area with a loud mitral first sound may indicate relative MS—relative because of the disproportion of the size of the valve and the ventricle. These murmurs disappear when the carditis disappears. The murmur of true MS is similar except that, in addition, early in diastole a snap is heard because of mitral valve opening. A later snap in diastole occurs with pericarditis and must be distinguished from the third heart sound.

Late signs are the blowing diastolic decrescendo murmur of AI, heard best with the diaphragm stethoscope just to the left of the sternum in the third interspace. This murmur may radiate down the left sternal border. A systolic high-pitched murmur in the third left interspace, with a decreased pulmonic second sound, is usually caused by PS.

Tricuspid murmurs are rare and are similar in character to mitral murmurs; a systolic murmur indicates tricuspid insufficiency, and a diastolic murmur indicates TS.

The murmurs heard in the tricuspid area and the murmur of PS are more often congenital than acquired during childhood. The murmur of AS is frequently caused by congenital lesion, and the murmur of AI is rarely heard during childhood, since AI develops late in the course of rheumatic carditis.

Venous hum is a continuous, low-pitched sound originating in the internal jugular vein, heard sometimes over the clavicles. It usually radiates downward and has no pathologic significance but must be distinguished from a murmur. The hum is usually louder when the patient is sitting, disappears in recumbency, may be abolished by pressure on the internal jugular vein, and is louder on the right. Venous hums over the abdomen, especially near the umbilicus, are sometimes heard in children with cirrhosis of the liver or portal obstruction.

Pericardial friction rub is a grating to-and-fro sound heard through the stethoscope as though it were close to the examiner's ear. It is increased by pressure of the stethoscope on the chest or by the patient leaning forward. Intensity of the rub varies with the phase of the cardiac cycle. Rub usually indicates pericarditis (e.g., tuberculosis or acute rheumatic fever), and sometimes may be detected on palpation as a vibratory thrill. Pleuropericardial rubs are more common than pericardial rubs and are heard best in the manner described, but they vary with the phase of respiration rather than with cardiac activity. They may be confused with pericardial rubs, usually have no pathologic significance, and may be caused by the proximity of the heart and lungs but may indicate pleuropericardial adhesions. Sometimes the crunch of subcutaneous emphysema is confused with a pericardial or pleuropericardial rub.

In general, type of heart disease is not diagnosed by examination alone. First, make a tentative diagnosis by history and repeated observation and try to confirm or eliminate this diagnosis by examination and suitable laboratory studies: For example, children aged less than 5 years rarely have rheumatic fever; even if aged more than 5 years, they should have other characteristic signs of rheumatic fever such as joint pains, subcutaneous nodules, chorea, or erythema nodosum. Even in older children without fever or increased pulse rate, a diagnosis of rheumatic fever is not very likely, although it is possible. If a child has fever, increased pulse rate, and murmurs, also consider the diagnosis of fever with innocent murmurs or myocarditis secondary to infection elsewhere, as in nephritis, diphtheria, or tonsillitis.

In children aged less than 5 years, next consider whether the heart disease is cyanotic or acyanotic. Severe cyanosis at birth, which has been determined (as described in Chapter 9) in a newborn to result from heart disease, usually indicates one of the most severe congenital heart lesions such as transposition of the great vessels, truncus arteriosus, or tricuspid atresia. Cyanosis developing later in the first year of life occurs because of an increasing shunt from the right heart to the left, such as in tetralogy of Fallot in which the increasing PS causes increasing right ventricular pressure. Cyanosis developing at age 4 or 5 years may indicate Eisenmenger complex or PS with septal defect. If cyanosis is not present unless the child exercises or cries, an atrial septal defect without PS is suggested because the right-sided pressure is not increased until the intrapulmonary pressure is increased by crying.

The significant noncyanotic heart diseases of infancy are toxic myocarditis from any cause, endocardial fibroelastosis, tumors of the heart, and, most commonly, PDA and coarctation of the aorta. Patent ductus arteriosus (PDA) has the characteristic murmur. In coarctation, pulse pressure is high in the arms and very low in the legs and femoral pulses are absent or weak. Other noncyanotic heart lesions, such as right aortic arch and dextroposition of the heart and aortic vascular ring, are diagnosed by examination and by history suggesting obstruction of the trachea or esophagus by an extrinsic mass.

The signs of heart failure in young children are not similar to those in adults. Early, the respiratory rate in the supine position is rapid; slight dyspnea follows. Next, the heart enlarges—best detected by scratch percussion. The liver becomes enlarged early and there may be venous engorgement and orthopnea; pulsus alternans and gallop rhythm, if present, are almost pathognomonic of heart failure. Signs of pulmonary or peripheral edema are noted late in the progression of heart failure as the failure becomes more severe. Sweating may occur.

The Abdomen

The abdomen is frequently examined first in younger children. The examination requires few instruments, but even they may frighten the child. Warm your hands before examining the abdomen. A thorough examination is impossible if the child is afraid or crying or if the abdominal wall is taut. Sometimes it is necessary to examine parts of the abdomen while the child is quiet and to examine the abdomen later when the child quiets again. If the child is ticklish, have the child place a hand over your palpating hand.

INSPECTION

First, inspect the abdomen, noting its *shape*. Ordinarily the abdominal musculature of children is thinner than that of adults, and children have a lordotic stance, giving the appearance of a "potbelly." This appearance can generally be considered normal until children reach puberty.

Real *distention* of the abdomen is usually caused by air or fluid in the bowel or peritoneal cavity, but it may also be caused by atonic abdominal musculature, paralysis of the abdominal musculature, feces in the bowel, abnormal enlargement of organs, intestinal duplication, or tumors. Distention is frequently noted in children with cystic fibrosis, celiac disease, hypokalemia, rickets, hypothyroidism, bowel obstruction, constipation, ileus, or ascites. Transilluminate the abdomen with a strong light beam to differentiate cystic from solid masses in a child with an enlarged abdomen. Transillumination helps detect cystic tumors, bladder distention, and multicystic or hydronephrotic kidneys, as well as ascites.

Respiration is largely abdominal in children until age 6 or 7 years; even after this age, the abdominal wall usually moves with respiration in children lying supine and in pregnant adolescents. Peritonitis, appendicitis, other acute surgical emergencies of the abdomen, paralytic ileus, diaphragmatic paralysis, a large amount of ascitic fluid, or a large amount of abdominal air may be present if the abdominal wall fails to move with respiration. If respiration is entirely abdominal in a young child or largely abdominal in an older child, suspect emphysema, pneumonia, or other pulmonary disorders.

The abdomen is normally flat when the child is in the supine position. Occasionally, however, the abdomen will appear depressed or scaphoid. In newborns this may signify a large diaphragmatic hernia with most of the abdominal contents in the chest. In older children, scaphoid abdomen occurs in cases of marked dehydration or high intestinal obstruction. With pneumothorax, the chest is large and the abdomen, although normal, may appear to be scaphoid.

Observe the *umbilicus*. Normally it is closed and puckered, but hernia may be present as observed by protrusion of some abdominal contents. Retraction of the umbilicus during voiding may indicate a urachal anomaly. Umbilical hernias are common in all infants until age 2 years and in black children until age 7 years. Hernias are especially common in children with hypothyroidism, Down syndrome, or the chondrodystrophies, or in large, chronically distended abdomens. Granulomas, ulcers, and drainage of the umbilicus occur in newborns and are discussed in Chapter 9. Umbilical hernias and diastasis of the recti can become obvious when the child cries or coughs. Paradoxical motion of the umbilicus is noted in unilateral or asymmetric paralysis of the abdominal wall musculature or of one part of the diaphragm.

Diastasis of the rectus muscles may be noted as a protrusion in the midline, usually from the xiphoid to the umbilicus but occasionally down to the symphysis pubis. Ordinarily the protrusion is one half to 2 inches wide; it is usually a normal variant but may be caused by a congenital weakness of the musculature or a chronically distended abdomen.

Note the *veins*. In infants with good subcutaneous tissue, veins are rarely visible. Visible but not distended veins are usual until puberty in healthy children and are especially noticeable in malnourished children. Veins are distended in heart failure, peritonitis, and venous obstruction. Milk a vein toward and away from the heart to determine direction of flow of blood in dilated veins. Blood flow from the veins below the umbilicus, normally downward, is usually reversed in children with obstruction of the inferior vena cava or portal hypertension (caput medusae). Diffuse epigastric pulsations may be normal or may indicate right ventricular hypertrophy with transmission of the pulsations through the diaphragm.

Next look for *peristalsis*, or *gastric waves*. Peristalsis is most easily seen if your eye is about at the level of the abdomen and a light is directed across the abdomen. Moving shadows will be noted in the presence of excessive peristalsis. Visible peristalsis is always a sign of obstruction until ruled otherwise. It may be seen normally in thin, small infants, especially premature ones. In infants aged 2 months or less, visible peristalsis may indicate pyloric stenosis or pylorospasm, but the type of obstruction cannot be distinguished by the nature of the visible peristalsis.

AUSCULTATION

Next, auscultate the abdomen and listen for peristalsis. It is better to auscultate the abdomen before proceeding not only because you may forget to listen if this part of the examination is postponed, but also because later manipulation may so alter peristaltic sounds that appraisal becomes inaccurate.

Peristaltic sounds are normally heard as metallic short tinkling. A sound may be heard normally every 10–30 seconds. Place the stethoscope firmly over the abdomen and listen carefully because the sounds may normally be of low intensity. You may cause sounds to increase in frequency and intensity simply by stroking the abdomen with a fingernail. The sounds are high-pitched and frequent in early peritonitis, diarrhea from any cause, intestinal obstruction, and gastroenteritis. Peristaltic sounds are absent in paralytic ileus. Listening to the abdomen and hearing the typical sounds of peritonitis may be the only way of detecting peritonitis in nephrosis or in other conditions in which there is free fluid in the abdomen, since free fluid may give you the impression of a nontense abdomen even though peritonitis is present. Rarely a venous hum may be heard during auscultation as a sign of portal obstruction. A murmur may be heard over the abdomen in children with coarctation of the aorta. Auscultate the area over the kidneys posteriorly with the bell stethoscope in children with hypertension. A murmur in this area may suggest constriction of one of the renal arteries.

PERCUSSION

After auscultating the abdomen, percuss by the indirect or scratch methods previously described. A tympanitic sound in a distended abdomen signifies that gas is present in the abdomen. Tympanites, or an unusually tympanitic sound, is common with low intestinal obstruction, air swallowing, and paralytic ileus.

A distended abdomen with little tympany suggests the presence of fluid or solid masses. When you suspect fluid, test for *fluid wave* and *shifting dullness*. Fluid wave may be elicited in the following manner: The edge of an aide's hand is placed firmly along the midline of the abdomen. Place one of your hands on one side of the patient's abdomen. Sharply strike the opposite side of the patient's abdomen with your other hand. A wave is felt against your first hand, as if the wave arises from deep in the abdomen. Shifting dullness is most easily obtained by percussing and delineating the area of dullness with the patient in one position. Then, change the position of the patient and elicit dullness again. Slight shifting dullness is normal or may be found with tumors, but considerable shift usually indicates free abdominal fluid. Fluid in the abdomen (ascites) is found in children with chronic liver disease (e.g., cirrhosis), chronic kidney disease (e.g., nephrosis), tuberculous peritonitis and, rarely, heart failure or rupture or other leak of the abdominal lymphatics (chylous ascites).

Solid masses will also be percussed. Frequently, a dull percussion note indicates a mass that cannot be felt. There is always dullness to percussion in the area of the liver unless free air is present in the abdominal cavity.

PALPATION

Several methods are satisfactory for palpating the abdomen, but in using all methods you should consider the comfort of the patient and yourself.

Distract the patient during abdominal palpation by making unrelated conversation or using other means. Palpating the abdomen with the child asleep is especially helpful if an acute abdomen is suspected. If the patient will cooperate, ask the patient to take deep breaths and to flex the knees during this part of the examination. Palpation is best performed if it can be done in inspiration and expiration. Place one hand flat on the patient's back and the other on the anterior surface of the abdomen. First, palpate gently and *superficially*, using the upper hand for most of the palpatory sensation. Begin in the left lower quadrant and then proceed to the left upper, right upper, right lower quadrants, and middle. If a localized site of pain or tenderness is found, palpate this area after the other parts of the abdomen have been palpated. Note first whether the abdomen is soft or hard. In a *tense* abdomen, there is a feeling of marked rigidity or resistance to pressure. A hard, tense abdomen immediately directs you to consider a surgical condition, any condition that may produce tenderness or, rarely, tetanus and hypoparathyroidism. In a crying child, distinguish between a soft and hard abdomen by feeling immediately on inspiration when the child may relax for an instant. This act may relax the abdomen enough to allow you to feel masses or to localize tenderness or rigidity.

Note *tenderness* and the point of maximal tenderness. Frequently a patient will say an area is tender, and you may doubt the accuracy of the statement. In such case, it is best to touch a completely neutral area such as the thigh and ask the patient if that area is tender. Do not ask the patient, "Does this hurt?" unless the patient is old enough to give a completely reliable response. Rather, you can determine the site of tenderness by watching the patient's face, noting wincing, cry, and change in pitch of cry as the actual tender area is touched. Note the patient's pupils when you palpate. When a truly tender area is touched, the pupils will dilate. Frequently, a child with pseudopain will keep the eyes closed during the examination, but with organic pain, the child will eye your hand as you palpate.

When asked where the abdomen hurts, a young child almost always points to the umbilicus. If the child points to any other part, pathology may be indicated. Tenderness can be further localized by noting pain on *rebound*. Place one hand deep in the abdomen, away from the suspected area of tenderness, and quickly remove your hand. The child may again complain of pain in the originally suspect area.

In general, even localized tenderness is not well correlated with underlying pathology. Tenderness in the lower quadrants may be due to such states as gastroenteritis, feces, obstruction, tumor or, rarely, Meckel diverticulum with ulceration, torsion of the ovary, and torsion of the testes. Lower abdominal tenderness after a menstrual period may result from pelvic infection. Tenderness in the right lower quadrant with exquisite superficial skin tenderness may be caused by appendicitis or abscess; in the right upper quadrant by acutely enlarged liver, hepatitis, cholecystitis, pelvic inflammation, or intussusception; and in the left upper quadrant by acute splenic enlargement, intussusception, or splenic rupture. Midline tenderness in the upper abdomen may result from gastroenteritis, coughing, vomiting, or gastric or duodenal ulcer. In the midline of the lower abdomen, you can distinguish marked superficial tenderness from muscle tenderness by asking the child to raise the head and then palpating. Intraabdominal tenderness is lessened, whereas superficial tenderness is increased by this maneuver. Disease in or near the spinal cord can cause referred pain to the abdomen.

Poorly Localized Abdominal Tenderness

Mesenteric adenitis	Peritonitis
Respiratory infection	Rheumatic fever
Sickle cell anemia	Measles
Allergy	Leukemia
Emotion	Acidosis
Pancreatitis	Ruptured viscus

If the abdominal wall is not tense, feel for the superficial masses. An enlarged *spleen* is usually felt as a superficial mass in the left upper quadrant. It may feel like a tongue hanging from the left costal margin, with a sharp straight border and a notch on the anterior margin. Splenic enlargement is evident in children with such diseases as septicemia; other infections; blood dyscrasias, including sickle cell or iron-deficient anemia; thalassemia major; hemolytic jaundice; infectious mononucleosis and leukemia; lysosomal storage diseases; and connective tissue diseases. A very large spleen with a less enlarged liver is evident in cases of portal vein obstruction and neonatal hepatitis. It may be normally palpable 1–2 cm below the left costal margin in newborns (because of extramedullary hematopoiesis) and in normal infants and young children. Note the size of the spleen and whether it is tender. Floating ribs are sometimes confused with the spleen on palpation. Usually you can differentiate by palpation or percussion.

The *liver* is generally palpable as a superficial mass 1–2 cm below the right costal margin, with a sharp border in newborns and infants. Ask older children or adolescents to breathe in and bring the liver edge down to your finger. Note size, consistency, tenderness, and pulsation. Throughout childhood, the liver may remain palpable without having pathologic significance.

Total span by percussion is about 5 cm at 6 months of age, 7 cm at 3 years of age, 8–10 cm at 10 years of age, and 9–12 cm at adolescence. If the span is larger or more than 2 cm below the costal margin, such states as passive congestion, hepatitis, tumor or metastases, blood dyscrasias, septicemia or other infections, reticuloendothelial or metabolic disease, or pulmonary emphysema may be indicated. A rapidly enlarging liver is an early sign of right heart failure. The liver edge is usually not as sharp in heart failure as it is in pulmonary emphysema without failure. Rapidly decreasing liver size may be diagnostic of acute liver necrosis. A thrill is felt over an enlarged liver or a gurgling sound is heard with hydatid echinococcal cysts in the liver. Friction rub over the liver usually results from transmission of the impulse from the aorta, but quite rarely it may result from tricuspid regurgitation or stenosis or constrictive pericarditis.

Other *masses* such as neuroblastoma, Wilms' tumor, duplication of the intestinal tract and urinary bladder, circumscribed collections of blood, collection of fluid in the uterus resulting from an imperforate hymen, hydrometrocolpos, and an enlarged uterus attributed to pregnancy may be palpated superficially. Push the spleen medially, laterally, and upward if necessary to distinguish it from an enlarged left lobe of the liver. It may be felt superficial to the colon, distinguishing it from a retroperitoneal mass. Wilms' tumor may be distinguished from a neuroblastoma, since Wilms' tumor ordinarily does not cross the midline; however, it may be bilateral, especially in younger children. Ovarian tumors palpated in preadolescent girls may be malignant; after menarche, they are more likely to be functional.

After palpating, superficially proceed in the same manner around the quadrants of the abdomen but palpate more *deeply*, using the posterior hand to push masses forward. The anterior hand pushes down so that the skin of the anterior abdomen is actually indented 2–5 cm. In children with ascites, it may be

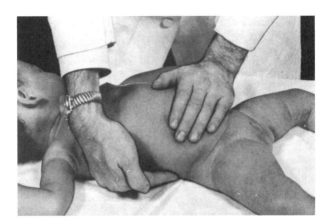

Figure 6-1.   Ballotting for right kidney.

difficult to feel any masses directly. However, percussion may indicate a few areas of increased dullness, and palpation by *ballottement* should delineate a few of the larger masses. In ballotting (Fig. 6-1), place one hand lightly above and one hand firmly below the area to be balloted. With the balloting hand, quickly flick the area. If a ballottable mass is present, a rebound sensation will be felt in the flicking hand, as if a ball had been thrown forward and came back.

In addition to delineating the masses felt on light palpation, look for deeper masses. For example, the tumor of pyloric stenosis is best felt on deep palpation after an infant vomits. This mass is usually located at the end of the stomach anywhere along the edge of the liver from the costal margin in the midline to the underside of the right lobe of the liver. The sausage-shaped tender mass of intussusception can usually be palpated in the right upper quadrant. Other masses such as those caused by urinary tract anomalies (e.g., malposition, hydroureter, and hydronephrosis) and the filled bladder may be palpated. *Bladder* enlargement may be attributable to anatomic urinary tract obstruction, voluntary control, embarrassment of the patient, or low spinal cord lesions.

By placing the index finger in the costovertebral angle and pushing up gently but sharply (as in ballottement), you can usually palpate about 1 or 2 cm of the right *kidney* and frequently the tip of the left kidney. The reverse procedure even more frequently allows you to feel the normal as well as the enlarged kidney: Gently elevate the abdomen of the child in the supine position with one hand, and place all the fingers of the other hand flat over the back of the elevated side so that the index finger lies in the costovertebral angle. Release the hand that is holding the abdomen forward; as the side of the abdomen falls toward the mattress, the kidney will hit the back of your hand. Enlarged kidneys usually indicate infection, congenital anomaly, tumor of the kidney, or renal vein thrombosis.

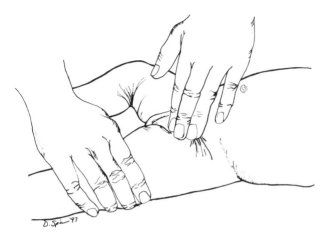

Figure 6-2.   Palpating femoral area for femoral pulse.

Remember that a few children have malrotation of the organs, as in situs inversus and congenital malrotation. In children who have had operations for repair of omphalocele and sometimes for diaphragmatic hernia, the organs are so displaced that it may be impossible to recognize even normal organs.

Every mass in the abdomen must be explained adequately before a patient can be considered free of disease. Occasionally, however, you may mistake feces in a child who is not even constipated for an abnormal mass or confuse the abdominal aorta with such a mass. Palpate the umbilical hernia previously noted. Note the presence of bowel in the hernia by palpating a gas-filled loop and obtaining the feeling of silk rubbing against silk on replacing the viscus. If the hernia cannot be easily reduced, make careful note of its size. Palpate also for a diastasis between the rectus muscles.

Obtain *abdominal reflexes* by scratching the skin of the abdomen with four scratches to make a diamond, the points of the diamond being the midline shortly below the xiphoid and above the symphysis and both sides of the abdomen at the level of the umbilicus. The umbilicus normally moves at each scratch. The upper scratches are innervated at T 7–T 9, and the lower at T 11–T 12. This skin reflex is absent in normal children aged less than 1 year and in children with early poliomyelitis, multiple sclerosis, or other central or pyramidal disorders.

Next, palpate the inguinal and femoral regions for hernias, lymph nodes, and femoral pulses (Fig. 6-2). *Femoral pulses* are best felt by placing the tips of two or three fingers along the inguinal ligament about midway between the iliac crest and symphysis pubis. With gentle pressure, you should feel definite pulsation with one of the fingers. Alternatively, pressure on the two or three fingers by the fingers of the other hand may make it easier to feel the pulse. Absent femoral pulse indicates coarctation of the aorta. Auscultation over the femoral artery may detect booming sound or "pistol shot," characteristic of AI or other causes of increased pulse pressure. A double sound (Traube's double tone) is indicative of the same conditions. A systolic and diastolic murmur may also be heard in these conditions (Duroziez's disease). Hernias are palpated as described below.

One of the favorite sites of determining *dehydration* in a child is over the abdomen. Pull up about 2 or 3 inches of the skin and subcutaneous tissue and quickly release it. If the creases formed by pulling the skin do not disappear immediately, dehydration exists.

Occasionally the wall of the abdomen feels puttylike in *consistency*. This may be normal, but it occurs in children who are chronically malnourished or dehydrated and in children with such diseases as peritonitis, tuberculous enteritis, the lysosomal storage diseases, myxedema, and hyperelectrolytemia.

GENITALIA

Inspect the genitalia. The mother of the patient or another woman should be in the room when you perform a vaginal examination. Answer succinctly any questions the patient raises. Inspect pubic hair, mons pubis, labia majora, labia minora, clitoris, urethral meatus, and vaginal introitus for presence, location, infestations, appearance, and discharge. A large clitoris (a glans wider than 10 mm) may be normal or an isolated physical finding; however, it may indicate adrenal hyperplasia or any of the conditions associated with precocious puberty defined as occurring before age 8 years in girls. The clitoris may not develop in adolescent girls with hypopituitarism or gonadal dysgenesis. The external genitalia grow very little until adolescence starts. In early puberty, a rectal examination and an examination with the girl on the examining table with the knees bent and the soles of the feet flat allows the patient to hold the labia apart. Show the equipment to be used and explain any expected pain or pressure. Pubic hair stages (Fig. 3-3) are useful in quantifying development. *Urethral discharges* are always pathologic in childhood and may indicate infection anywhere in the urinary tract. A flaming red area around the end of the urethra may be caused by prolapse of the urethral mucosa. Eccentric masses near the urethra may be cyst, urethral polyp, papilloma, caruncle, condyloma, sarcoma botryoides, prolapsed ureterocele, or periurethral abscess.

Inspect the vaginal orifice (Figs. 6-3 and 6-4) with the girl in the knee-chest position. In preschool and primary school girls the opening is about $1-4 \times 3-8$ mm; in preadolescent girls, it is about 1–2 mm larger. Rough vaginal borders or an orifice larger than 1 cm in diameter may indicate manipulation or abuse. Small tender ulcers may be indicative of herpes simplex or other infections, including other sexually transmitted diseases.

Adhesions of the labia majora in a newborn may be a congenital malformation or may occur in children with congenital adrenal hyperplasia. Imperforate hymen may be noted; this may cause hydrocolpos in young girls or hematocolpos in pubertal girls. Have the patient cough. With imperforate hymen, the hymen bulges. With absent vagina, the vaginal area is retracted upward and the hymen does not move. Vaginal septa may cause similar signs. The labia minora are prominent in newborns, then

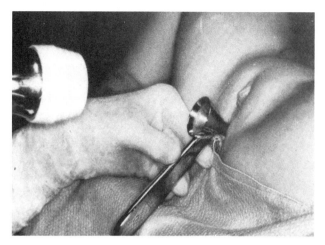

Figure 6-3. Inspection of the vagina with a vaginoscope for children and simple illumination with a flashlight.

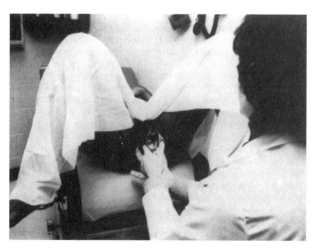

Figure 6-4. Proper draping for pelvic examination.

atrophy, and are virtually absent until estrogens are produced at adolescence. Adhesions of the labia in older girls may be caused by infections, irritation, or local trauma, including abuse, and may cause dysuria.

A bloody *vaginal discharge* is normal but not common up to the fourth week of life and at menarche. Vaginal bleeding in children aged less than 8 years is usually attributable to foreign bodies, injury, or constitutional isosexual precocity; ovarian tumors, botryoid sarcoma, and carcinoma of the cervix may present similarly. A mucoid vaginal discharge is frequently noted. In children still in diapers this usually results from irritation caused by the diaper or the powder used in the diaper region. In older girls a foul discharge may be due to tight panties or pants, intertrigo, masturbation, pinworms, infection secondary to a foreign body, or allergy. A thin watery discharge is common in girls for 2–3 years before onset of menstruation. Redness of the perineum may be caused by irritation of physical or chemical agents such as bubble baths but may also signal a urinary tract infection. Discharge accompanied by red inflammation in the surrounding vaginal and urethral structures usually indicates disease. A white, practically odorless discharge has no significance.

A purulent discharge may be attributable to gonorrhea. Profuse, frothy, foul-smelling pruritic discharges may be due to *Trichomonas* organisms. White adherent discharge suggests *Candida* infection.

Foreign bodies are usually palpated by rectal examination. Urethral caruncle or *prolapse* of the urethra may be noted.

Vaginal palpation is usually omitted until near puberty. Note vaginal discharge or foreign body, size of uterus, and presence of ovaries. The normal uterus measures 1–2 cm, and the ovaries measure 0.5–1.0 cm until puberty. In older girls, use the lithotomy position with stirrups. Palpate the vaginal orifice before inserting the warmed speculum. Feel for enlarged glands, a sign of sexually transmitted infectious diseases. Do not lubricate the speculum before insertion, since this precludes obtaining cultures. Use a vaginoscope with a 1- × 11-cm blade. Press down on the introitus with one finger, insert the blade vertically, and then turn it horizontally; open it slowly with most pressure posteriorly. Maneuver the speculum until the cervix is seen. Do not stretch the hymen. Regardless of findings, do not use terms to describe the uterus such as *small, infantile,* or *underdeveloped,* since these terms may frighten the patient. The normal ratio of fundus to cervix is 1:3 in infants, 1:1 in pubertal girls, and 3:1 in mature women.

The cervix is normally pink and smooth, but columnar epithelium may extend over the junction, resembling erosion. The color becomes blue during pregnancy. Tenderness on moving the cervix or in the area of the fallopian tubes suggests pelvic inflammatory disease. An adnexal mass may be abscess, ectopic pregnancy, endometriosis, or ovarian cyst. An enlarged uterus occurs with intrauterine or ectopic pregnancy. Observe the vaginal wall for discharge or ulcers. Take cultures of any discharge, and endocervical swab for Papanicolaou (PAP) smear. Remove the speculum slowly. Proceed with bimanual examination; rectal examination is discussed below. Cover the gloved index and middle fingers with sterile lubricant and press posteriorly. Note any firmness or masses in the vagina. Note whether the cervix is firm or soft and whether the os is open or closed. Palpate the uterus between the abdomen and vagina: note its size, shape, and position and whether it is soft, firm, smooth, or tender. Palpate the adnexa on either side for enlargement, tenderness, or masses. The size of the ovaries normally is less than 1 cm before puberty and as much as 3 cm at puberty, and they may not be palpable unless they are enlarged.

Average adolescent development in girls proceeds as follows: breast development after age 8 years, pubic hair development at about age 12 years, increase in height velocity at age 12 years, and menarche and axillary hair before age 13 years.

In males, make a note if the position of the urethral orifice is not at the tip of the glans. *Hypospadias* exists if the opening is on the ventral (inferior) surface, and *epispadias* exists if the opening is on the dorsal surface of the penis. Examine the prepuce for infection, posthitis, and *phimosis* (a small opening of the prepuce). Some adhesions of the prepuce to the glans are normal until about age 4 years. Foreign body may be felt as a hard mass in the urethra. The prepuce may be inflamed, swollen, and tender. Inflammation of the glans (balanitis) may cause urinary obstruction. Pink pearly papules (1- to 3-mm elongated papillae on the corona of the penis) are normal in adolescents. Venereal warts are less uniform in size. Herpes simplex may resemble a small tender pimple, whereas a syphilitic chancre is a larger, less tender ulcer.

An enlarged penis may be noted in children with precocious puberty, CNS lesions, some testicular tumors, and adrenal hyperplasia. In congenital adrenal hyperplasia, the penis is large but the testes are of normal size. The penis may appear small if it is obscured by fat in corpulent boys. The penis is small in adolescent boys with hypopituitarism.

Observe the *meatal* opening. Stenosis may cause the opening to appear round instead of slitlike. Ulcers may cause obstruction to urinary flow. Note strength of stream. Slow stream indicates obstruction.

Next look at the *scrotum*. Normally the scrotum of a child who is not cold or frightened is loose and the testes and cords can be felt in it. Anything else in the scrotum is abnormal. If the scrotum appears large, suspect hernia or hydrocele or both. Often, especially in premature infants, the scrotal sac appears small, empty, and underdeveloped. Make an inverted "V" with your index finger and thumb together, place them about half an inch above the center of the inguinal ligament, and gently push toward the scrotum. Somewhere along the inguinal canal, a soft mass will be felt. Then try to push this mass into the scrotum. Once the mass is in the scrotum, grasp the mass with the thumb and forefinger of the opposite hand. If it can be brought to this position even though it may immediately retract, the mass is normally descended *testis*. Repeat the procedure on the opposite side. If the mass is palpable in the inguinal canal but cannot be pushed down or if the testis is not felt, suspect an undescended or abdominal testis. In an older boy, one maneuver to bring the testis down is as follows: Have the boy sit in a chair with his heels on the seat, grabbing his knees. The extra abdominal pressure may push the testis into the scrotum. A small, flat, underdeveloped scrotum is probably the most accurate indication of true maldescent (cryptorchidism), usually resulting from defects in the inguinal canal but possibly signaling hypogonadism.

The testes are smooth; their size is usually about 1 cm until puberty. At stage II of puberty, testes' length is 2–3.2 cm; at stage III, it is 3.3–4.0 cm; at stage IV, it is 4.1–4.9 cm; and at stage V, it is 5 cm. They remain small in children with hypopituitarism. They are large in boys with fragile X syndrome and are uneven and enlarged with infection or tumor of the testis. They are large with precocious puberty, defined as occurring before age 9 years in boys, but not with precocious puberty secondary to adrenal hyperplasia. A hard, enlarged testis without pain suggests tumor.

Average penile length as measured with a ruler at the base of the gently pulled penis is 4 cm at birth, 5 cm at age 4 years, 6 cm at age 11 years, and 12 cm at the end of adolescence. Micropenis is found in children with chromosome abnormalities, Prader-Willi syndrome, and other dysmorphic syndromes. If the penis is normal or small and the testes are firm and small in the adolescent, gonadal dysgenesis (Klinefelter syndrome) may be present. The left testis is usually lower than the right; the opposite may indicate complete situs inversus.

If the scrotum appears large, changes size, or enlarges with coughing or crying, place one finger on the external inguinal ring and palpate the scrotum. If the mass in the scrotum feels firm, it is probably normal testis. If something is palpated in addition to the testis and cord, try to determine whether the sensation obtained is that of fluid, gas, or solid structure. Try to reduce the mass in the scrotum by pushing the contents back through the external ring. Masses that cannot be reduced include incarcerated hernia, hydrocele, varicocele, and spermatocele, in addition to normal structures.

Next, shine a light through the mass. If the mass (except the testis) transilluminates and is irreducible, fluid is probably present. If the mass does not transilluminate and is irreducible, hernia is probably present. The use of transillumination in young children may be misleading because bowel in a hernial sac may transilluminate.

If a bulge occurs in the inguinal canal, and if a mass that is neither testis nor fluid is found in the scrotum, or you have the sensation of gas (crepitus) on palpation, the patient has a visible *hernia*. If you feel crepitus when you try to push the mass through the external ring, hernia is likely. Tenderness may be noted. In contrast to hydroceles, hernias are usually tender. Next, auscultate over the scrotal sac. Peristaltic sounds help indicate the presence of a hernia.

Hernias that cannot be reduced despite careful manipulation are said to be *incarcerated*. Hernias that feel swollen or have become gangrenous are *strangulated* from the tight constriction of the neck of the sac.

Finally, if a hernia or hydrocele is suspected, feel over the internal ring with the flat part of the index finger and roll the spermatic cord beneath the fingers as it lies in the inguinal canal. Although the ring is normally open, only a thin 1- to 2-mm solid structure should be felt extending through the ring. If the cord feels thickened or like silk being rubbed on silk, peritoneum is going through the ring, denoting a hernia that may be invisible. The size of the structures in the canal can be determined and thickened structures may indicate polyarteritis, hernia, or other abnormality. Occasionally a hydrocele of the spermatic cord can be felt and may be mistaken for an incarcerated hernia. Careful palpation of the mass helps separate the upper end of the hydrocele from the internal ring, which is not possible with a hernia.

If an observer reports the presence of a hernia but none is found, the following maneuvers may make the hernia obvious: Have the patient stand on the examining table, and place the flat of your hand on the patient's abdomen. Pump the abdomen in and out with several short frequent strokes, and the hernial sac will become apparent. An older child may sit on a stool and hold the knees while you try to straighten the legs. The hernial sac will then fill.

Fluid in the scrotum usually indicates the presence of a *hydrocele*. Hydroceles are found frequently in children aged less than 2 years, are usually not tender, and with closed tunica vaginalis testis usually do not change size when reduction is attempted. Fluid fluctuating in volume denotes the presence of a patent tunica vaginalis testis or indirect inguinal hernia. *Varicocele* feels like a "bag of worms" because of the dilation of the pampiniform veins and usually occurs on the left. *Spermatocele* is a benign cyst on the head of the epididymis.

Acute *swelling* of the scrotum with discoloration may occur in those with Mediterranean fever or may result from torsion of the spermatic cord, a surgical emergency. Acute painful swelling also occurs in boys with orchitis, epididymitis, Henoch-Schoenlein purpura, or rarely, torsion of the testis appendages. With torsion, the testicle is higher in the scrotum than it should be and may appear to lie transversely. With epididymitis, the testicle is in the normal position, and the long axis usually is in the axis of the body. The spermatic cord is tender and swollen with epididymitis and tender but not swollen with torsion. Elevation of the swollen tender mass decreases the pain in epididymitis and increases the pain with torsion. Epididymitis is usually caused by infection and accompanied by signs of urethral infection, but it may be a presenting sign of sarcoid. The testis may be dislocated into the inguinal canal after trauma.

Differential diagnosis of testicular torsion, incarcerated inguinal hernia, epididymitis, and orchitis—all of which cause scrotal swelling—may be difficult. With testicular torsion, the spermatic artery on the involved side does not pulsate. Pulsation is increased with orchitis, epididymitis, and torsion of the testicular appendix. Orchitis is usually accompanied by mumps or other viral infection.

The *cremasteric reflex* is tested by stroking the inner aspect of the thigh. The testis will rise in the scrotum, sometimes rising into the canal. This reflex is normal at any age. Absence may indicate a low spinal cord lesion, as in poliomyelitis, or testicular torsion but it is also frequently absent in normal boys, especially at age less than 6 months and age more than 12 years.

Examine the *lymph nodes* in the inguinal region for size and tenderness. Ordinarily three or four 0.5- to 1.0-cm glands are not abnormal. Tenderness or enlargement always indicates infection or any of the systemic diseases associated with generalized enlarged nodes.

The average adolescent development in boys proceeds as follows: testicular enlargement at age 11.5 years; pubic hair, development at age 12.5 years; increase in height velocity at age 14 years; and development of facial and axillary hair at age 14.5 years.

ANUS AND RECTUM

Examine the anal region; however, rectal examination is not performed in a routine examination but is reserved for children with symptoms referable to the lower gastrointestinal tract or those with abdominal pain.

Observe the *buttocks* for masses and firmness. The intergluteal cleft should be straight. Deviation occurs with sacrococcygeal tumor in the buttocks or hip dysplasia. Masses over the coccygeal area are usually sacrococcygeal tumors. Tufts of hair, meningocele, pilonidal dimple, and perianal abscess may be noted. If a pilonidal dimple is present, carefully inspect it for presence of a sinus. Abscesses may be caused by *rectal fistula*. Therefore, determine the extent of any rectal fistula by observation and probe if the full extent of the fistula cannot be visualized.

The buttocks are usually firm, even in advanced malnutrition; however, in cystic fibrosis and celiac syndrome, they are flattened. The skin creases of the buttocks are usually asymmetric but may indicate the presence of congenitally dysplastic hips. Skin creases of the buttocks are especially prominent in children with recent weight loss.

Anal fissure appears as a cut or tear in the mucosa. It is one of the most frequent causes of constipation or rectal bleeding in infants until age 2 years and may cause infantile "colic." Anal fissure is best detected by placing the infant on the abdomen, pulling the buttocks apart, and noting the fissure and asymmetry of mucosal folds. This maneuver may cause bleeding.

Note prolapse of the rectal mucosa. It may be a cause of infantile colic. It may be caused by chronic constipation, straining, severe coughing, or diarrhea and may occur with cystic fibrosis or neurologic or anatomic abnormalities.

Note other *protrusions* from the anus. Small mucosal tabs have no significance; however, cherry-red, round protrusions may be rectal polyps and cause rectal bleeding. Solid dark protrusions are hemorrhoids. They may be caused by portal hypertension, and may cause profuse bleeding. Large flat tabs of skin may be condylomas, a sign of papilloma virus infection, syphilis, or sexual abuse.

Pinworms occasionally are noted in the perianal area in the folds of rectal mucosa; these may cause rectal itching. A dark *ring* around the rectal mucosa may be an early sign of lead poisoning.

Most of the eruptions around the rectum in the young result from diaper rash. Usually the eruption is a generalized reddened or brawny area with vesicles or papules. However, pustules may be present and represent secondary infection of the diaper rash or perianal cellulitis resulting from streptococcus or candida.

A *rectal* examination is best performed with the infant or child lying supine with the legs flexed. A child who is old enough is asked to empty the bladder before this examination. Ordinarily, your fifth finger is long enough to provide the required information in infants and hurts the patient less than a larger finger. Because you may have better control and mobility of the index finger, use it for more precise information. Grease the anus and finger cot well before inserting your finger. Imperforate anus is evident immediately, since the finger cannot enter beyond the dimple.

Note sphincter *tone*. A patulous rectum is associated with sexual abuse or a low cord injury, including myelomeningocele and diastematomyelia. A tight sphincter is generally a developmental variation indicating stenosis. Anal stenosis may cause constipation and pain on defecation. A rectovaginal *fistula* exists if your finger enters the vagina through the rectum.

Occasionally, you will feel a shelflike protuberance 2–5 cm above the anus; this, with absence of feces in the rectum, may be a sign of aganglionic megacolon. Anterior position of the anal opening with a posterior shelf on rectal examination is a sign of anterior ectopic anus, a cause of chronic constipation. If position is uncertain, measure in girls from fourchette to anus to coccyx and in boys from the base of the scrotum. The distance of fourchette or scrotum to anus divided by fourchette or scrotum to coccyx is 0.39 or 0.56, respectively. Marked deviation indicates displacement.

The anus and rectum may be distended with feces in children with mental delay, chronic constipation, or psychogenic difficulties. Absence of feces in the rectum in an acutely ill child may indicate ileus, peritonitis, or obstruction.

Note masses. Fecal masses of any consistency can be removed. A tender mass in the lower quadrants may be found with a low intussusception. A right lower quadrant mass is occasionally noted with acute appendicitis or appendiceal abscess and sometimes with regional ileitis. Polyps may occasionally be felt in the rectum. Masses that displace the rectum forward frequently are teratomas. Other masses described under examination of the abdomen are also noted.

Palpate for the *prostate*, a flat mass several centimeters up and on the midline anterior wall of the rectum. Any prostate that is larger than 1 cm before age 10 years may indicate precocious puberty or congenital adrenal hyperplasia. After puberty, the prostate is 2–3 cm and is smooth. A tender prostate indicates infection; an uneven or large prostate suggests tumor.

Rectal examination is also useful in palpating the *uterus*. In pubertal children and occasionally in younger children, the ovaries may also be palpated. The prepubertal uterus is felt as a 1- to 2-cm oval mass anterior to the rectum and about 3 or 4 cm above the symphysis pubis. When the ovaries are palpable before puberty, they are about 0.5 to 1.0 cm in diameter, situated about 2–3 cm laterally and just above the uterus. Foreign bodies in the vagina or rectum can also be felt by palpation.

Even though a rectal examination is usually uncomfortable and is reserved for the last part of the physical, it can frequently localize tenderness in the abdomen. After your finger is well up in the patient's rectum, place it in the midline and press the other hand toward the finger. Note facial expression. Next, move the finger and the abdominal hand to the left, and repeat on the right. Differences in facial expression or rigidity of the lower abdomen is a clue to abdominal or rectal pathology.

Sensation should be tested in children who are suspected of having a spinal cord lesion or a patulous rectal sphincter. Use a pin to touch the perineal region at closely approximated points. Twitching of the perineum normally occurs with a slight lateral movement of the anus. Absence of this reflex suggests lower motor neuron lesion.

If you wish to visualize the rectal mucosa for suspected internal rectal fissure, polyp, hemorrhoid, colitis, proctitis, or bleeding site, you may do so with relative ease with a small proctoscope or without special equipment. Grease a clean test tube and push it

Stool Color	
Brown, yellow	Normal
White	Acholic, excess milk ingestion
Bright red (blood)	Anal fissure, lower colon
Bright red (not blood)	Foods, dyes
Black, tarry (blood)	Bleeding proximal to ileocecal valve

about 5 cm into the rectum. Place a small light just behind your shoulder, shining into the tube. Slowly withdraw the tube, and note the mucosa as it falls back into place. Note the color of the stool (see box).

Extremities, Joints, and Spine

In practice, the physician usually examines the extremities, bones, joints, and muscles simultaneously and then, if abnormalities are detected, examines the systems under suspicion individually and more extensively. Examination of muscles is described in Chapter 8.

The order of examination of these systems depends largely on the age, condition, and cooperation of the child. If the child walks, make preliminary observations of posture, gait, and stance immediately. Note the position the child assumes during the examination either during this part of the examination or as part of the general appearance of the patient. For teenage atheletes, a brief examination is helpful (Table 7-1).

EXTREMITIES

In patients aged 2–6-years, you may begin the physical examination with observations of the hands and feet. Most children at this age are happy to show their hands and feet when requested and are especially happy to see no instruments present at the beginning of the examination. Persistently pink hands and feet are a sign of poor nutrition, poor hygiene, or other types of deprivation.

Infants who hold both their arms immobile in 90-degree flexion at the elbow when lying, sitting, or standing may be suffering from emotional deprivation. Infants who appear to look at one arm for a long time or who hold one arm in an unusual position for 1 or 2 minutes may have infantile autism. Such posturing is normal until about age 6 months. Stereotypic hand movements and hand wringing in young girls may be a sign of Rett syndrome or autism.

Note congenital *anomalies* of the arms, hands, legs, and feet. These include amelia (absence of the part), webbing, and extra digits.

Length and shape of the extremities are usually determined by nutritional and congenital factors. Abnormalities (e.g., long, thin extremities) are noted in children with arachnodactyly. Broad, short extremities are noted in children with Down syndrome, mucopolysaccharidoses, or chondrodystrophies. Apparent shortening of the thumb and fourth and fifth fingers occurs almost always in children with pseudohypoparathyroidism.

Shortening of an extremity is usually congenital but may result from disease of the epiphyses or cerebral palsy. Inequality of leg length may be present in children after femoral fractures or with dislocation of the hip or other hip disorders.

Lengthening of an extremity is usually congenital but may result from large hemangiomas, lymphangiomas, arteriovenous fistula, neurofibromatosis, or hemihypertrophy. Generalized enlargement of the extremities may result from any of these factors and, when unilateral, may cause hemigigantism. Enlargement may also be attributable to lymphedema praecox or congenital lymphedema (Milroy disease), as a manifestation of ovarian dysgenesis, Turner syndrome, or edema.

Table 7-1.   *The 2-minute orthopedic examination*

Instructions	Observation
Stand facing examiner	Acromioclavicular joints, general habitus
Look at ceiling, floor, over both shoulders	Cervical spine motion
Shrug shoulders (examiner resists)	Trapezius strength
Abduct shoulders 90 degrees (examiner resists at 90 degrees)	Deltoid strength
Full external rotation of arms	Shoulder motion
Flex and extend elbows	Elbow motion
Arms at sides, elbows 90 degrees flexed; pronate and supinate wrists	Elbow and wrist motion
Spread fingers; make fist	Hand or finger motion and deformities
Tighten (contract) quadriceps; relax quadriceps	Symmetry and knee effusion; ankle effusion
"Duck walk" four steps (away from examiner with buttocks on heels)	Hip, knee, and ankle motion
Turn back to examiner	Shoulder symmetry, scoliosis
Keep knees straight, touch toes	Scoliosis, hip motion, hamstring tightness
Raise up on toes; raise heels	Calf symmetry, leg strength

Reproduced from *Sports medicine: health care for young athletes*, Elk Grove, IL: AAP, 1983.

Inspect fingers and toes for *clubbing* (hypertrophic osteo-arthropathy) (Fig. 7-1). Elevation of the nail base is an early sign of clubbing. Later, the entire end of the finger, including the nail region, appears expanded and rounded as compared with the remainder of the finger. Ask the child to oppose both thumbnails. A small diamond-shaped opening is normally visible. With club-bing, no space is present. Clubbing may occur in any condition of reduced circulating oxygen, such as cyanotic congenital heart disease or chronic pulmonary disease, and also in patients with chronic liver disease or bacterial endocarditis. Clubbing may be a presenting sign of cystic fibrosis, Crohn's disease, ulcerative colitis, celiac disease, gastroesophageal reflux, intestinal para-site infestation, and thalassemia. Unidigital clubbing may be due to phalangeal bone lesions such as in sarcoid.

Pain and *tenderness* in the extremities are usually caused by trauma or infection. Pain, especially of the legs, is noted in infants with scurvy. Infants aged less than 3 months with con-genital syphilis may have pain causing pseudoparalyses. Tenderness over the sartorius muscle may be noted in children with tuberculous meningitis. Tenderness elicited at a point in the bone by sharp percussion of the distal end of the bone sug-gests the presence of osteomyelitis (Fig. 7-2). Inability to supinate the hand with the arm held in flexion and pain in the elbow indicates subluxation of the head of the radius.

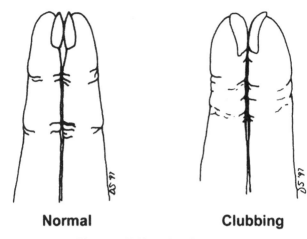

Normal   **Clubbing**

Fig. 7-1. Clubbing (described in text).

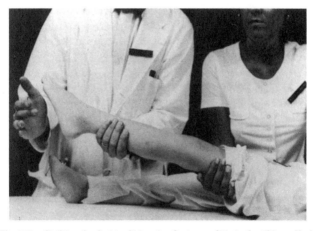

Fig. 7-2. Striking the foot to elicit pain of osteomyelitis in the tibia or fibula.

Pain in the knee or foot may result from local disease, but it also requires examination of the hips. Pain in the knee that increases with internal rotation of the tibia may be caused by osteochondritis dissecans. Pain in a bone that is worse at night and is rapidly relieved by aspirin is characteristic of osteoid osteoma.

Note the *temperature* of the extremities, taking special care to note whether the temperature is equal bilaterally. Differences in temperature are usually attributed to neurologic or vascular abnormalities. Cold, pallid extremities may occur after sympathetic nervous system stimulation or may be a manifestation of venous or arterial thrombosis or embolism. With nervous system lesions, pulsations are usually present, whereas with vascular lesions pulsations are usually diminished or absent.

Necrosis of the extremity, or *gangrene*, may result from obliteration of the vascular supply. The area is cold, avascular, pallid, and tender, with loss of muscle power. The area may gradually become black and less painful as necrosis proceeds. It may ooze and be moist and obviously infected or it may be dry. Gangrene may develop in infants after embolism, particularly from the umbilical venous system; after severe trauma or infection to the part; and sometimes after frostbite.

Enlargement of the bones may be caused by infection in the bone. Swelling with joint tenderness, heat, and redness near but not in the joint is characteristic of osteomyelitis. Swelling may result from periosteal hemorrhage, as in scurvy; from cortical thickening, as in congenital syphilis, vitamin A poisoning, or infantile cortical hyperostosis; from localized increased calcification, as in callus formation after fracture or in rickets; or from bone cysts or tumors. Auscultation over the area of the swelling may reveal a bruit, more common in osteomyelitis than in the other causes of increased vascularity of the bone.

Enlargement of the tibial tubercles with tenderness is characteristic of Osgood-Schlatter disease, probably from stress on the patellar tendon.

Bony, painless swelling at the epiphysis adjacent to the knee or wrist joints is one of the most definite signs of rickets. Symmetric swelling of both hands or both feet in infants may indicate the hand–foot syndrome of sickle cell anemia.

Other *deformities* of the bones are usually caused by fractures. Fractures are evidenced by the patient's inability to use the limb, by deformity, or by excess motion in the bone with pain and crepitation. Auscultating at the proximal epiphysis while tapping the distal end of a bone elicits a difference in sound on the nonfractured side from sound elicited on the fractured side. Fractures are almost always caused by trauma and may suggest child abuse. Multiple fractures may result from polyostotic fibrous dysplasia, bone cysts, other diseases of the parathyroid gland, prolonged bed rest, or osteogenesis imperfecta.

Note *shape* of the bones. Lateral bowing of the tibia (genu varum) is present when the child stands with the medial malleoli in apposition, and a persistent space more than 2 cm is observed between the medial surfaces of the knees. Frequently infants are bowlegged for 1 year after starting to walk. Significant genu varum may result from anomalies of the feet or from rickets. Anterior curvature of the tibia may indicate congenital syphilis. Excess bowing just below the knee may indicate osteochondrosis deformans, Blount disease, or tibia vara.

Knock-knees (genu valgum) can be determined when, with the knees together, a child's medial malleoli persistently are separated more than 2 cm. Knock-knees are usually normal in children from about 2–3½ years of age. Knock-knees may also be evident in children with pronated feet, rickets, or syphilis.

Bony hard enlargement of the medial or external aspects of the femoral or tibial epiphyses is usually a normal variant but may occur with rickets or other metabolic bone diseases or with dysgenesis of the knees such as dysplasia epiphysialis hemimelia.

Tibial torsion, a twisting of the tibia probably initiated by the intrauterine position, is best determined with the patient on the back and the knees facing upward. Both the forefoot and the hindfoot will be held in a plane but not in line with the knees. With the tibial tubercle and the patella in a straight line, place your fingers on the malleoli. In infants, the line joining the four malleoli should be parallel to the table. In older children, as much as 20 degrees of external torsion is normal. With any greater deviation, or if the lateral malleolus is anterior to the medial malleolus, inward tibial torsion may be present. With fixed deformities of the foot such as metatarsus varus, the forefoot will be adducted in this position but the hindfoot will be in a straight line with the patella.

Note the *feet* for abnormalities. At birth, the child's feet are usually held in varus or valgus attitude—almost never straight. An easy method to determine whether this position, which is the intrauterine position, will straighten is simply to scratch first the outside and then the inside of the lower border of the foot. In self-correctable deformities, the foot will assume a right angle with the leg. More severe anomalies, such as clubfeet or metatarsus varus, either can be straightened only by forceful manual stretching or cannot be straightened by manual means at all (Fig. 7-3).

Because all children have a fat pad under the arch, the feet may appear flat until the child has walked for 2 years. A very high-arched foot (pes cavus) may be noted in some normal children or in patients with Friedreich ataxia or in various lower motor neuron lesions. Talipes equinus, with short heel cords and weightbearing on the toes, may be characteristic of cerebral palsy or muscular diseases; it results in spasm and contracture of the muscles of the leg and may cause "toe walking." Many normal children walk on their toes until age 3 years.

Toe walking may also indicate muscle imbalance, spasticity, muscular dystrophy of the Duchenne type, or disorders causing weakness of the peroneal and anterior tibial muscles. Children with septic arthritis of the hip walk on their toes to relieve strain around the hip. Some autistic and some normal children also toe walk.

Examine the heel cords with the patient in the supine position and the knee extended. Grasp the foot by the heel (Fig. 7-4), with the sole lying in your hand; slightly invert the foot to lock the heel and then dorsiflex it. Tight cords are present if dorsiflexion cannot be carried to about 20–30 degrees beyond a right angle.

Note pronation of the feet. Pronation becomes apparent when the child stands. A pronated foot is flexible and may appear normal when the child lies on the table, but it will abduct at the forefoot when the patient stands, with obliteration of the long arch, bulging of the medial border of the foot, and outward angulation of the forefoot on the hindfoot. The medial malleolus may appear closer to the floor than normal, there may be knock-knees, and the thighs may appear adducted. The weight-bearing line, which is the line through the middle of the patella perpendicular to the floor, will cross the inner border of the foot instead of going through the second toe as is normal. From the back, the heel cord, which normally descends perpendicularly, will be noted to curve outward with eversion of the heel (valgus heel).

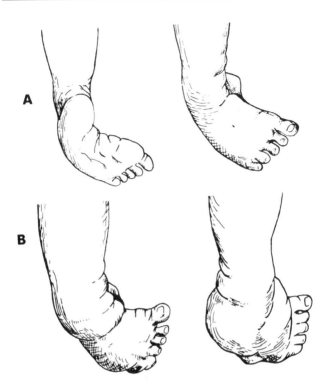

Fig. 7-3. A: Forefoot adduction; heel inversion. B: Talipes equinovarus.

After examining the feet, look at the patient's shoes. Abnormal wear or misshapened shoes may help you to diagnose gait or foot disorders. Then note the patient's *gait* and *stance*. Observing the child in a room with a mirror at one end is helpful when studying the child's gait. Observe the anterior and posterior aspects simultaneously as the child walks toward and away from the mirror. The child should be wearing shoes or at least socks, because bare feet on a cold floor may distort the gait.

Normally a child aged 1–2 years walks with a broad-based gait, frequently with the hands out to the side. Gradually as the child reaches the age of 3 or 4 years, the legs are brought together and the toes are straight ahead. An older child with a broad-based gait may have abnormal mechanics of the legs or feet or may use this gait for balance if normal neural positioning and balancing mechanisms are defective. Watch for truncal ataxia as the child turns. Ask children aged more than 3 years to walk on their toes to demonstrate distal muscle weakness, a sign of peripheral neuropathy. Ask children aged more than 4 to walk on their heels. Asymmetry suggests mild hemiparesis or hemiplegia. Ask children aged more than 5 to walk a line, heel to toe. Failure suggests a midline cerebellar lesion, a cerebellar tract defect, or gross motor incoordination.

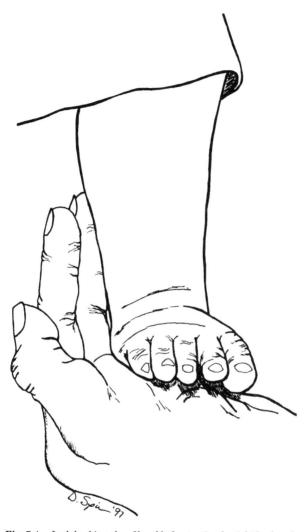

Fig. 7-4. Lock heel in palm of hand before testing for tight heel cords.

Balance, at rest or while walking, is maintained by normal cerebellar function, normal vestibular nerve function, and good muscle, bone, and joint functions. Loss of balance may be attributed to cerebellar or vestibular disease or muscle weakness. Deviation to one side during walking may indicate cerebellar disease of that side; lack of normal swing of the arm of that side suggests cerebellar or corpus callosum involvement.

Toeing in (pigeon-toe) or toeing out may be noted. Children with pronated feet may toe in or toe out. Other orthopedic conditions causing toeing in include internal rotation of the hips, tibial torsion, and metatarsus adductus.

A scissors gait with stiff crossing over of the legs as the child walks is evident especially in children with a spastic type of cerebral palsy or with mental delay. You can elicit this type of gait even in 7-month-old children if they are made to walk by being gripped under the shoulders and pushed along (Fig. 7-5). A wad-

---

Causes of Limping in Children

Skeletal System
  Trauma, fracture
  Foreign body
  Tumor
  Infections
  Postinfectious

Joints
  Synovitis
  Arthralgia
  Arthritis; rheumatoid,
    Kawasaki disease,
    Lyme disease, septic,
    parvovirus
  Dislocated hip
  Slipped capital femoral
    epiphysis
  Collagen vascular disease
  Henoch-Schoenlein
    purpura
  Legg-Calvé-Perthes
    disease, aseptic
    necrosis,
    Osgood-Schlatter
    disease
  Toxins
  Urticaria
  Foot injuries
  Bursitis

Nervous System
  Neuropathic conditions
  Central

Spinal Conditions
  Spondylitis
  Diskitis
  Epidural abscess

Muscular System
  Strain
  Sprain
  Myositis
  Myopathic conditions

Hematologic and Oncologic Conditions
  Sickle cell disease
  Leukemia
  Neoplasms
  Hemophilia
  Serum sickness
  Epstein-Barr virus

Intraabdominal Conditions
  Appendicitis
  Infection
  Inflammatory bowel
    disease
  Ovarian tumors, torsion
  Pelvic inflammatory
    disease
  Testicular tortion
  Inguinal hernia

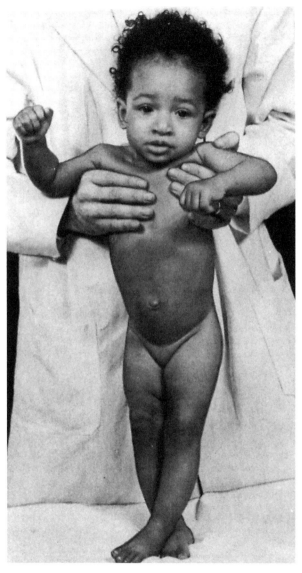

Fig. 7-5. Scissors gait can be demonstrated before child can walk by grasping under axillae and pushing patient forward.

dling gait may be noted in patients with bilateral dislocation of the hip or with coxa vara.

Note a *limp* of any type. A limp may result from local infection; muscle, nerve, bone, or joint disease; or pain, but it is most commonly caused by trauma, fatigue, or a pathologic condition of the hip. Pain in the foot, ankle, knee, hip, or spine requires careful examination of all five areas because pathologic conditions of the hip or spine may be referred to the foot or knee. Children with intraabdominal inflammatory disease (e.g., appendicitis, abscess, and retroperitoneal fibrosis) may limp.

You can examine young children who limp while they sit in the parent's lap. Observe the back, hips, buttocks, and extremities. Compare the gluteal folds; look for asymmetry, swelling, and erythema of the two sides. Palpate for induration, warmth, tenderness over bones, muscle spasm, and effusion or distention of the joint capsules of the hip, knee, and ankle. Test each joint for motion, examining the suspect limb or joint last. Note restriction of flexion, extension, abduction, adduction, and rotation. Measure limb girth and length. Perform rectal and neurologic examinations.

Limp occurs with soft tissue injury anywhere in the lower extremity. Soft tissue injuries include *sprains* and *strains*. Abnormal laxity of a ligament after injury associated with local pain is characteristic of sprain; swelling occurs because of bleeding into the joint. Disruption of a muscle–tendon unit is a strain. Similar signs may be noted in cases of epiphyseal fractures and dislocation of the patella. Foreign bodies, myositis, cellulitis, hives, bruising, and other lesions in the soft tissue may cause a limp.

JOINTS

Examine the joints for *heat, tenderness, swelling, effusion, redness*, and *limitation* or *pain* on motion. Redness, heat, and tenderness—signs of infection—are detected by observation and palpation. Effusion in the joint, a sign of any type of joint irritation, can be best determined by ballottement of the joint or by tapping on one side of the joint and feeling protrusion on the other side as a fluid wave is elicited. In children, the most common cause of tenderness in one joint with limitation of motion but without other physical signs is synovitis of traumatic or nonspecific origin.

Swollen, hot joints are seen in children with arthritis, hemarthrosis, or osteochondritis. Motion is limited in these conditions, usually because of pain and spasm of the overlying muscles and tendons. Arthritis of rheumatic fever is painful without much swelling and responds to aspirin more rapidly than rheumatoid arthritis in which the joints are stiff.

In rheumatic fever and systemic lupus erythematosus (SLE) the swelling may be reducible (Jaccoud syndrome). Pain in the joint without physical findings is arthralgia and may be caused by any condition discussed previously or by strains or overactivity.

Limitation of joint motion without pain may occur as a congenital malformation. Flexion deformities of the fingers and toes are common. Children with multiple congenital dislocations, as in arthrogryposis, may have severe flexion deformities of many joints. Limitation of joint motion is also common in children with various spastic neurologic disorders (described in Chapter 8).

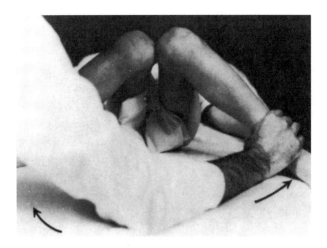

Fig. 7-6. External rotation of the hips.

Recurrent Joint Pain

Juvenile rheumatoid arthritis
Poststreptococcal arthritis
Parvovirus; other viruses
Rubella
Seronegative enthesopathy
   (SEA) syndrome
Reflex sympathetic dystrophy
Fibromyalgia
Rheumatic fever

Lupus erythematosus
Allergic reactions
Kawasaki disease
Hypermobility syndromes
General debility
Amyotonia congenita
Down syndrome
Ehlers-Danlos syndrome

Detect excess joint motion by hyperflexing or hyperextending the joint. Such excess motion usually results from relaxation of the structures surrounding the joint. Most children with chorea and children with rickets or malnutrition have hypermobility of the joints, especially of the wrists, because of poor muscle tone. Hyperextension of the knees (genu recurvatum) may be attributed to the intrauterine position, or may be evident in children with spina bifida, arthrogryposis, agenesis of the patella, or other malformations.

In infants, investigate the *hips* routinely for congenital dysplasia. With the infant on the back, flex the legs at the knees and attempt internal and external *rotation* by holding the knees and simultaneously rotating the thighs (Figs. 7-6 and 7-7). See whether the rotation is equal on both sides. Unequal rotation is usually caused by decreased mobility of one joint. The hips can be abducted and externally rotated so that the knees touch the tabletop in most infants. With unilateral subluxation, abduction is limited on the affected side (Fig. 7-7). A "click" heard after this maneuver may either be normal or a sign of dysplasia. Grasp the outer aspect of one thigh with the middle finger over the greater

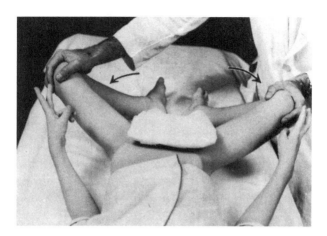

Fig. 7-7.   Internal rotation of the hips. Note that angles made by each leg are equal.

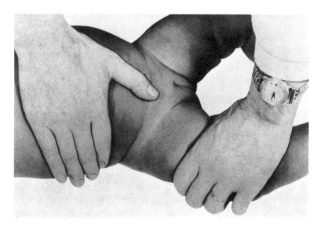

Fig. 7-8.   Piston mobility. Grasp thigh firmly.

trochanter. Lift and abduct the thigh. A "clunk" indicates that a dislocated hip has been reduced (Ortolani click).

Determine *piston mobility* in children with hip joint dislocations by holding the hip region with one hand, grasping the thigh with the other hand, and pulling the hands apart gently (Fig. 7-8). Motion that occurs as in a Slinky toy is piston mobility. A little motion, possibly as much as 1 cm, is normally present, but with congenital dysplasia the hip motion may have a range of 2 to more than 2 cm below the socket. As the child grows older, tightness of the adductor muscles is noted, and the *gluteal folds* may be uneven. Normal children may have uneven gluteal folds.

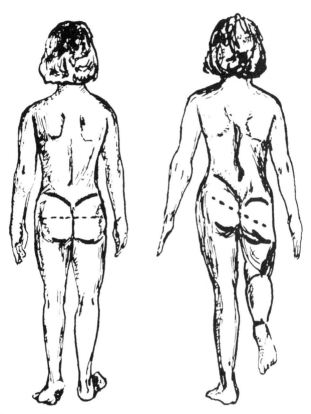

Fig. 7-9. Trendelenburg sign. When the child stands on both feet, the pelvis is level; when the child stands on the affected side, the normal side drops.

In addition to recognized congenital dysplasia, older children, especially those who are obese, may have progressive subluxation of the hip. The child with dislocation of the hip usually has a painless limp with apparent shortening of the leg on the involved side. When the child is asked to stand on the normal limb and raise the other leg, the pelvis on the involved side rises to maintain balance. When the patient is asked to stand on the leg with the dislocated hip and raise the normal limb, the abductor muscles cannot raise the pelvis and it drops (Trendelenburg sign) (Fig. 7-9). A painless limp, worse with fatigue, occurs also with coxa plana, especially in boys.

A painful limp with limited motion especially in the morning is usually evident in children with tuberculosis of the hip. In addition, in this disease, the hip is first abducted and later adducted with flexion on the pelvis. If it appears that children are simulating limps or abnormal gaits, tell them to run, touch a spot, and return. Usually they will concentrate on your instructions and forget to simulate.

Limited motion of the *elbow* with weakness after injury suggests tennis elbow. Pain is felt over the lateral epicondyle because of strain. In the child aged less than 2 years, inability to supinate the hand with the arm held in flexion, along with pain in the elbow, indicates subluxation of the head of the radius.

Tenderness of the tip of the *ankle* malleoli after injury suggests fracture.

Knee Injuries

Examine the unaffected knee first, with the patient in the supine, sitting, and standing positions. Note angular deformities, the presence of effusion, ecchymoses, abrasions, scars, and gait if weightbearing is possible. With the knee extended, try to push fluid from the outer to the medial side of the joint with the flat part of your hand. A bulge of the synovial lining, particularly on the medial side of the knee, indicates effusion. Transillumination will help you recognize the presence of fluid. Check for muscle atrophy of the thigh or calf. Check range of motion (ROM) last if effusion is present. If effusion occurs shortly after injury, suspect a serious injury with hemarthrosis. Delayed onset of effusion after injury suggests strains or an inflammatory process. Limited flexion or extension of the knee with a limp may result from dislocation or chondromalacia of the patella (peripatellar bursitis) after injury, osteochondritis, other bone disease, or all other joint diseases.

Palpate to identify the site of maximum pain. Pain in the joint suggests a cartilage or ligament injury. Stress the joint by abducting and adducting with the patient in the supine position and with 30-degree flexion. Pain elicited in a patient in the supine position suggests medial ligament injury; at 30 degrees, it indicates collateral ligament injury. Test with 90-degree flexion, pulling on the proximal tibia. Excess displacement indicates cruciate ligament tears.

Flex the hip and knee and rotate the foot. A click indicates a torn meniscus. Locking of the knee suggests intraarticular loose bodies. Pain in the tibial tubercle suggests Osgood-Schlatter disease resulting from bursitis or fracture. Pain or dislocation of the patella may indicate fracture. If the patella is not palpable, suspect peripatellar bursitis.

Shoulder Injuries

Compare both shoulders of the patient. Asymmetry may result from edema, deformity, trauma, septic arthritis, or osteomyelitis. Squaring of the shoulder suggests dislocation. Prominence of the distal clavicle may be attributed to acromioclavicular separation. A double bulge on the anterior surface of the upper arm when the elbow is flexed suggests rupture of the biceps tendon. Note the point of maximum tenderness and try to identify the part of the joint, tendon, muscle, or bone involved. Have the child fully abduct the arm to locate limitation. Pain and paresthesia radiating from the shoulder to fingertips relieved by shoulder elevation suggests referred pain from cervical radiculopathy. Atrophy of the deltoid muscle suggests axillary nerve injury. A prominent scapula with painful muscles suggests rotator cuff injury.

SPINE

Examine the patient's spine in routine physical examinations. Observe infants in the supine position. The infant may kick and move during the examination. Then place the infant on its abdomen. In older children, make observations with the patient in the sitting or standing position. Note the way the child stands or walks.

Tufts of hair, dimples, hemangiomas, discolorations, cysts, and masses are frequently seen near the spine. A tuft of hair over a small dimple in the midline usually indicates the presence of an underlying spina bifida or may simply be an ectodermal anomaly. Spina bifida occulta can occasionally be determined by pressing carefully over the suspect area when the trunk is flexed. The spinous processes above and below the spina bifida will feel thin and well formed, whereas the spinous process of the defective vertebra may feel split.

A small dimple in the midline anywhere from the coccyx to the skull may indicate a dermoid sinus. These dimples are important to record as possible entry points of infection to the central nervous system (CNS). Any of these may be associated with tethering of the cord.

Palpate and transilluminate *masses* over the spine. Nontender masses of varied color and consistency with a thin covering are usually meningoceles. Meningoceles, which communicate with the CNS, can usually be distinguished from noncommunicating masses by palpation. If signs of increased intracranial pressure such as bulging of the fontanel are apparent, it is likely that the contents of the mass communicate with the spinal canal. Cystic masses that transilluminate may be teratoma, meningocele, or lipomeningocele. Nontender, noncommunicating masses near the spine are usually lipomas or fibromas. Soft masses that feel like lipomas, usually with skin dimples, may also extend into the CNS and are lipomeningoceles.

Tender masses not communicating with the spinal canal are usually infectious and include tuberculous spondylitis and tuberculous and perinephric abscesses. Deep tenderness over the spine is usually caused by trauma of the spine or surrounding structures. Localized spine tenderness is best elicited by punching with the side of your hand or by tapping with the reflex hammer. Masses covered by skin over the sacrum or coccyx may be teratomas. These are firm and can usually also be felt on rectal examination.

Localized Back Tenderness

Cord tumor	Spondylitis
Injury, bone or muscle	Spondylesthesis
Diskitis	Stress fracture
Disk injury	Lumbosacral strain
Osteoarthritis	Spinal stenosis
Rheumatoid arthritis	Scoliosis
Hyperlordosis	

Examine the spine for intrinsic *motion*. Limitation of flexion is easily demonstrated by asking patients to sit up from a prone position. Patients with flexion limitation will turn over and maintain the position of the back with pokerlike rigidity. If patients are sitting, ask them to kiss their knees to demonstrate limitation of forward bending. If you place your fingers on several of the patient's adjoining spinous processes, the processes normally will move separately as the patient bends the trunk laterally. With stiffness of the spine, your fingers move as a unit.

The spine is stiff in children with CNS infections, especially meningitis or tetanus; in diseases or anomalies of the bones such as osteomyelitis of the spine, epiphysitis of the vertebrae, or hemivertebrae; or in patients with adjacent lesions such as peritonitis or perinephric abscesses. Occasionally, with severe trauma to the back, the spine will be rigid. Causes of limitation of motion of the spine in adults, and sometimes in adolescents, are protruding intervertebral disc and lumbosacral strain. Severe pain and tenderness over the spine, particularly at night, may result from a tuberculous abscess or cord tumor. Inflammatory disease or a tumor of or near the spine may cause referred pain to the abdomen, hips, knees, or legs.

Limitation of motion of the neck by muscle spasm is a prime neurologic sign of nervous system disease and is discussed in the section on other lesions of the neck. Nonneurologic causes of limitation of motion of the neck include rheumatoid arthritis of the cervical vertebrae; adjacent infections such as cervical adenitis and retropharyngeal abscess; rotatory subluxation of the cervical vertebrae; fracture or congenital anomalies of the vertebrae, especially hemivertebrae; or shortening of the sternocleidomastoid muscle producing torticollis (wryneck).

Excess mobility of the spine is rare and is most easily demonstrated with the patient in the supine position. Place one hand beneath the patient's head and the other under the knees. As the spine is flexed, it feels unusually supple, and the knees may easily approximate the chin. Such excess mobility is evident in those states that produce generalized hypotonia and is sometimes noted in small children with acute potassium deficiency.

Winged scapulae occur when the lower borders of the scapulae extend out loosely from the back, with excess mobility. Mild degrees occur often, but marked winging may be attributed to weakness of the muscles around the scapula. This weakness may occur after injury to the long thoracic nerve, in the muscular dystrophies, or in congenital anomalies such as absence of the clavicle (cleidocranial dysostosis) and high scapula with webbed neck (Sprengel deformity).

Note *posture*. Lordosis and kyphosis are exaggerations of the normal anteroposterior (AP) curvatures of the spine. Lumbar lordosis is normal in children throughout childhood and mimics the appearance of children with a protuberant abdomen. Marked lordosis may be caused by rickets, muscular dystrophy, or weakness of the abdominal wall. Adolescent round back is noted in children with chronic poor posture and thoracic epiphysitis.

Kyphosis is a sharp anteroposterior angulation of the spine opposite in direction to lordosis. It is usually caused by small or collapsed vertebral bodies. It is evident in cases of tuberculosis of the spine, but it may be a diagnostic sign of mucopolysaccharidosis, Morquio disease, or aseptic necrosis of the vertebral bodies. Localized kyphosis (gibbus) is caused by disease of one or two

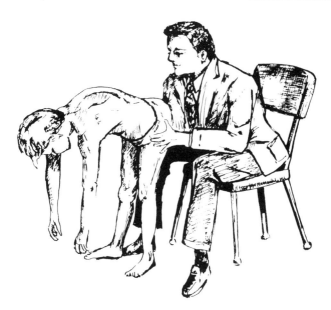

Fig. 7-10. Having a patient bend forward is the fastest way to detect scoliosis. The ribs rise. (Adapted from Netter F. *CIBA Clin Symp* 1978), 30:16.

vertebral bodies and may occur in the same disease states causing kyphosis. Lack of normal thoracic kyphosis may thrust the heart anteriorly (*straight back syndrome*).

Detect *scoliosis*, a lateral curvature of the spine. Scoliosis is detected by having the patient stand erect. Mark the tips of the spinous processes with ink. Note the deviation of these ink spots from a straight line when the patient stands upright while barebacked or in a plain tight-fitting top. Ask the child to bend forward with the knees straight and the arms hanging down. Structural scoliosis exists when (a) there is a double curvature with rotation (twisting) on the convexity, (b) the ink line does not straighten when the patient bends forward, or (c) one hip appears prominent. Note scapular asymmetry resulting from cervical or thoracic curves. Posterior ribs should be symmetric. A lump of one group of ribs indicates structural scoliosis (Fig. 7-10).

Mild scoliosis usually has no rotation, straightens in the prone position, and is related to poor postural habits. Scoliosis in a child aged less than 5 years is usually attributed to congenital anomalies or to lung or chest pathologic conditions. In older children, scoliosis may be idiopathic or caused by a difference in leg length, hemivertebrae, rickets, poliomyelitis, muscular dystrophies, or neurologic disorders such as neurofibromatosis. Some curving of the lower spine is evident in children with acute abdominal pathologic conditions such as appendicitis or pyelonephritis. Painful scoliosis, which is relieved by aspirin, is suggestive of osteoid osteoma.

Neurologic Examination

Neuropsychiatric examination is important both in examination of children who are not acutely ill and, because the central nervous system (CNS) is one of the common sites of infection, in acutely ill infants. In addition to careful observation and neurologic examination, a detailed history of the child's development and behavior is essential to the neurologic evaluation. Examination of the neck, a critical site of neurologic abnormality in an acutely ill child, is described in Chapter 4.

Neurologic examination of children differs from that of adults because the neurologic lesions usually sought in children differ from those in adults. For example, poisonings, congenital malformations of the brain, progressive brain diseases, and infections are common in children, whereas local vascular lesions are rare. Acute brain injury may be present in both children and adults, but bleeding in the brain of children may be accompanied by delayed onset of signs because of the distensibility of the skull. In children, as in adults, metabolic diseases may also often cause CNS signs. At the conclusion of the neurologic examination, you should have a good evaluation of the child's mental status and speech, cranial nerves, muscle coordination and control, and reflex sensory and autonomic functions.

Perform the neurologic examination, except assessment of such overall procedures as the mass reflexes, along with the general physical examination of each particular part of the body. Described herein are only the mass reflexes, the reflexes noted in the extremities, and general aspects of the neurologic examination. However, the neurologic examination may be repeated as a whole after the general physical examination—especially if any variants are detected or if neurologic difficulties are suspected—and may be recorded separately.

More important than examination of reflexes (except in children who are acutely ill with a neurologic disorder) is the *general impression* you have of the patient's *abilities* and *responsiveness*.

Although older children and adolescents may be examined in a manner similar to that used for adults, infants and younger children are examined largely by observation of the characteristic *positions* of the patient, the *spontaneous movements*, and the *play activity*. Some of these qualities are discussed in Chapters 3 and 7. To elicit this information, use not only patience but also imagination in your approach to younger patients. Especially in infants, compare motor and social accomplishments with suitable developmental charts (Appendix B), which with full realization of the wide variability of normal infants, helps indicate neurologic adequacy.

Note the *state of consciousness*, a combination of awareness and arousal. The patient may be hyperirritable, convulsive, hyporeactive, delirious, stuporous, or comatose. State of consciousness may be difficult to quantitate. Responses to commands, speech, name, pinprick, or severe pain are some of the usual tests for degree of consciousness. Lack of response, in the above order, indicates decreasing consciousness and increasing

Table 8-1. *Glascow Coma Scale*

Eye opening	Verbal	Motor	Score
		Follows commands	6
	Oriented	Localized pain	5
Spontaneous	Confused	Withdraws from pain	4
To speech	Inappropriate words	Abnormal flexion	3
To pain	Nonspecific sounds	Extension	2
None	None	None	1

a Add one number for each activity. Numbers 13–15 correspond to drowsiness; 10–12 to stupor, 7–9 to light coma; 4–6 to deep coma; and 3 flaccid and apneic. The scale is useful for following progression and regression.

stupor or coma. In deep coma, a patient's respirations, blood pressures, and reflexes are depressed (Table 8-1). Coma with focal signs and increased reflex activity is usually caused by a brain lesion; coma with multifocal signs and decreased reflexes is usually caused by metabolic disease or poisoning. Touch the child's eyelash lightly on either side with no warning. The child with feigned coma responds with a vigorous bilateral blink.

Generalized hyperirritability with hyperactivity in a child is usually a sign of psychologic difficulty. You can frequently elicit this response by observing the patient make quick movements when asked, for example, to draw a picture. Irritability may, however, be prominent in any ill child.

Hyperirritability—Hyperactivity

Fever
Hypoglycemia
Hyponatremia, hypocalcemia
Pain
Chalasia with esophagitis
Central nervous system
  disorders
Cardiac, pulmonary,
  intraabdominal
Other metabolic disorders

Hernia
Corneal abrasion
Hair around toe, finger, penis
Acrodynia
Scurvy
Collagen-vascular diseases
Chorea
Hyperthyroidism

Hyperactivity may be a cardinal sign of attention deficit hyperactivity disorder. Ordinarily, younger children will be more irritable when lying on the bed or examining table than when in their mothers' arms because of a natural fear of the unfamiliar surroundings. Some infants will be more irritable when in their mothers' arms. This *paradoxical irritability* should alert you to the possibility of CNS infections, particularly meningitis, although other disease states such as acrodynia, scurvy, severe febrile illness, fractures, and emotional disturbances may also manifest this sign.

Convulsive states are signs of disease and should never be considered diagnoses. Seizures manifest themselves in different ways. Record the type of seizure, the parts of the body involved, and seizure duration.

International Classification of Epileptic Seizures

Partial Seizures
    Simple partial (consciousness retained)
        Motor
        Sensory
        Autonomic
        Psychic
    Complex partial (consciousness impaired)
        Simple partial, followed by impaired consciousness
        Consciousness impaired at onset
    Partial seizures secondarily generalized

Generalized Seizures
    Absences
        Typical
        Atypical
    Generalized tonic-clonic
    Tonic
    Clonic
    Myoclonic
    Atonic
    Infantile spasms

Unclassified Seizures

Partial simple seizures are focal with normal consciousness and may be motor or sensory. Complex partial seizures (psychomotor, temporal lobe) may be characterized by alterations in consciousness and abnormal motor activity. Generalized seizures may be completely incoordinate tonic and clonic movements in unconscious children and may be caused by abnormal cortical discharges. Absence (petit mal) seizures are brain disturbances causing loss of consciousness for 5–15 seconds and are also accompanied by abnormal electrical brain discharges. Autonomic manifestations may consist of bizarre visceral disturbances and usually last longer than 30 seconds, followed by impaired consciousness, hallucinations, total amnesia, confusion, headache, and sometimes incontinence.

Most childhood seizures begin on one side and may be considered focal, but they quickly become generalized and the etiology is usually that of a generalized seizure. The causes of the irritability may include many types of metabolic, vascular, or CNS disorders. Seizures do not usually occur in children with brain tumors until the intracranial pressure is considerably increased.

Distinguish seizures from simple fainting (syncope). The latter is a sudden loss of consciousness without abnormal movements and is usually caused by reflex vascular disorders.

Syncope

Orthostasis	Aortic stenosis
Vasovagal tone	Cardiomyopathy
Vasodepressor	Anomalous coronary artery
Supraventricular tachycardia	Hyperventilation
Long QT	Drugs
Complete atrioventricular block	Psychogenic
Sinus bradycardia	

Seizures must also be distinguished from hysterical "fits," which are usually not accompanied by injuries or other neurologic signs and may contain periods during which the hysterical child is responsive. They must be distinguished from exaggerated startle response with falling followed by hypertonia and ataxia, hyperekplexia. Syncope that occurs with the child on a table tilted 60–80 degrees for 30 minutes helps indicate neurocardiogenic causes. Syncopal episodes occur suddenly; they may result from cardiac dysrhythmias with no premonitory sensation. They occur more commonly when the child is sitting, standing, or coughing. Seizures can occur when the child is lying down or when the child has cardiac dysrhythmias, mitral valve prolapse, gastroesophageal reflux, migraine, or Tourette syndrome. Seizures resulting from vagal-mediated cardiac arrest can be produced by 10 seconds of pressure on the eyeballs. Seizures preceded by crying or cyanosis are commonly associated with breath-holding.

Lack of total activity, demonstrated by the persistence of one position for long periods, is common in mentally or emotionally delayed children or may be a sign of severe debility, malnutrition, or anemia. Catatonia, in which one unusual or apparently uncomfortable position is assumed for a long time, may be seen in mentally delayed or psychotic children. Catatonialike observation of the finger and hands is normal in the 3- to 6-month-old child.

Lack of all activity is usually caused by a state of unconsciousness—stupor or coma—and must be differentiated from normal sleep states from which the patient can easily be aroused.

In older children, look for other neurologic evaluation before the reflexes are elicited. Note the patient's gait, stance or limp, as described in Chapter 7.

Note *ataxia* as gross incoordination. Brain tumors, especially of the cerebellum, and encephalitides may be accompanied by ataxia. Ataxia caused by sensory or proprioceptive loss is worse with the eyes closed. The general weakness characteristic of the amyotonias, dystrophies, or spasm of the muscles of the thigh in hip disease is sometimes mistaken for ataxia. Other cerebellar injuries, such as cerebral palsy with cerebellar involvement, the degenerative ataxias, some CNS infections, or tick paralysis, are especially likely to be followed by ataxia. Ataxia worsened by heat occurs in multiple sclerosis. Ataxia may occur as nonepileptiform seizures. A variety of drugs, including phenytoin, phenobarbital, and the antihistamines, may cause ataxia in sensitive persons. Vestibular damage, as is sometimes manifest in children treated with streptomycin, may be followed by ataxia.

Note *coordination*. Incoordination may be caused by cerebellar lesions or by any of the diseases that cause ataxia. Watch the child reach for a toy, tear paper, tie shoes, and button a shirt. Coordination is easily tested by playing a game with the child. Sit opposite the child with the child's palms upward and ask the child to strike first your right and then your left hand. Continue at a rapid pace, and then shift the position of your hands. Inability of the child to follow the motion of the hands may indicate varying degrees of incoordination.

Coordination may also be tested by the finger-to-nose or heel-to-shin tests in the child who can understand commands. In these tests, tell the patient to extend first one hand and touch the tip of the nose with the index finger. The patient then repeats the action with the opposite hand, usually after you demonstrate. Then tell the patient to repeat the same procedure with the eyes shut. Gross incoordination is the failure of the patient to touch the nose with the eyes open. Minor evidence of incoordination, as well as lack of sense of position, will be manifested by the patient's inability to perform these tests with the eyes shut. Remember that fine coordination is not fully developed in children until 4 or even 6 years of age, and if a younger patient can bring a finger within 3 or 4 cm of the tip of the nose, coordination is generally considered normal.

Have the patient perform the heel-to-shin test by running the heel of one foot down the anterior aspect of the tibia of the other foot. Usually you also demonstrate this to the patient. A child's inability to perform this test is a less reliable guide to evidence of incoordination or lack of position sense in a child, but results of tests with the eyes open and shut are similar in significance to those of the finger-to-nose test. Fear and anxiety may result in apparently poor coordination. When asked to jump rope, some anxious children will demonstrate superior coordination and balance when jumping rope with both feet or with one foot and even with the eyes closed. Ask the child to hop. Inability to hop after age 5 years indicates lack of gross motor coordination.

Note *tremors* and distinguish them from choreiform movements (Table 8-2). Tremors are constant, small movements; some occur when the patient is at rest because of lesions of the extrapyramidal system, and some occur only when voluntary motion of the part is attempted (intention tremor). Intention tremors result from lesions of the cerebellum. Tremors in the infant are seen with states of hypocalcemia and hypoglycemia. Muscular tremors or fibrillations may be noted when certain muscles are fatigued and in children with hyperthyroidism, hypothermia, hyperthermia, or progressive degeneration of the cord. Most commonly, tremors or twitchings occur in infants in bursts, without obvious cause.

Table 8-2.   *Involuntary Movements*

Type	Character
Athetosis	Slow, continuous, writhing
Chorea	Random, jerky
Dystonia	Slow, twisting mingled with muscle tension
Fasciculation	Coarse twitching
Fibrillation	Rapid twitch in muscle
Hemiballismus	Flinging, jumping, wild, unilateral
Jack-knife	Body bends at waist (see myoclonic)
Myoclonic	Sudden, brief, shocklike
Myokymia	Twitching of muscle fibers
Spasm	Prolonged muscle contraction
Tardive dyskinesia	Writhing, fibrillation of tongue and face
Tics	Involuntary muscle contractions, noises, words
Tremor	Fine or coarse shaking
Twitch	Spasmodic, short

Twitchings (tics) are spasmodic movements of short duration, noted in muscles that are fatigued in which a nerve is regenerating, that occur in children with chorea. Movements stop during sleep. In contrast to children with dyskinetic movements or dystonia, children with chorea do not lose consciousness. Twitchings may occur after sharp pain in an area. In emotionally upset children, the twitchings follow a definite and usually periodic pattern. In children with Tourette syndrome, the twitchings increase in frequency and the children develop vocal bursts.

Choreiform movements are coarse, involuntary, purposeless movements associated with decreased muscle tone. They are quick, jerky, and irregular, grossly incoordinate, and movements may disappear with relaxation. In chorea associated with rheumatic fever, movements may involve any muscle, including those of the tongue, speech, hands, and feet. These movements are best elicited by having the patient extend a hand or perform other voluntary acts. The fingers and wrists will hyperextend, and the choreiform movements of the fingers become exaggerated. With extension of the arms above the head, the palms of the hand point outward and the hand is flexed at the wrist with extension of metacarpal and interphalangeal joints. Choreiform movements are also noted in patients with hereditary ataxias, lupus erythematosus and with drug reactions. Choreiform movements may be one-sided (hemichorea) and, in rare cases, are caused by vascular brain lesions (hemiballismus). Paroxysmal choreoathetosis occurs after startle, lasts less than a minute, and recurs several times a week; the cause is unknown.

Athetosis refers to a group of constant, gross incoordinate movements that are slow and writhing and are usually associated with increased muscle tone. These movements are exaggerated by voluntary activity and disappear when the patient relaxes during sleep. *Dystonia* is a slow, twisting movement of limbs or trunk. Athetosis usually indicates basal ganglia involvement; ataxia and incoordination occur with even superficial cerebellar lesions. Athetoid movements may occur in children with cerebral palsy or tuberous sclerosis and are present late in the deteriorating course of the reticuloendothelial diseases such as Niemann-Pick and Tay-Sachs. Infants may normally have athetotic movements during their first year of life.

A periodic nodding of the head (spasmus nutans) resembles athetosis. It may be idiopathic, may occur as a habit spasm, or may be a sign of mental deficiency, tumors near the optic chiasm or third ventricle, neuroblastoma, or gastroesophageal reflux. The nodding is a combination of true anteroposterior nodding and lateral shaking, which may be temporarily interrupted by suddenly attracting the child's attention. Infants with spasmus nutans usually also tilt the head and have nystagmus. To-and-fro motions of the head synchronous with the pulse (Musset sign) may occur in cases of aortic insufficiency.

Note *associated* movements—voluntary movements of one muscle accompanied by involuntary movements of another muscle—regulated by the cerebellum. They occur as mirror movements in the Klippel-Feil syndrome, in diseases with increased intracranial pressure, and in patients whose handedness has been changed. Reciprocal movements occur normally in infants aged 2–4 months and usually decrease by age 4–6 months; failure of these movements to appear or disappear at the proper times is an indication of brain damage. Certain reciprocal movements such as the movement of the arms when a person walks are normal at all ages, and their absence may indicate cerebellar damage or absent corpus callosum.

Note handedness by observing the preferential handling of small objects. Definite handedness in a child aged less than 15 months suggests hemiparesis.

Note the muscles for *development, tenderness, spasm*, and *paralysis*. Muscle *tone* is caused by a balance between muscle mass and nerve stimulation. It represents the degree of contraction in the voluntarily relaxed muscle. Test muscle tone by grasping the muscle or pressing on the muscle and estimating its firmness; watch the muscle response during its normal ROM with and without resistance, such as response to painful stimuli in the region activated by the muscle. Assess muscle strength of an older child by having the child perform against resistance supplied by your hand.

Muscle tone is increased in any condition causing muscle spasm. Muscle spasm is felt as unusual tenseness of the muscle mass and may occur in injury or infection of the muscle, bone, or joint; in metabolic disease; or in children with upper motor neuron lesions. Muscle spasm is also noted in diseases affecting the spinal cord roots, probably secondary to pain. Spasm occurs in overused muscles, in myositis due to bacterial or viral infections, toxins or, occasionally, before pain, as in children with tumors of the cauda equina or in patients with abnormalities of the filum terminale, who manifest hamstring spasm early.

Generalized spasm may be evident early, involving almost all striated muscles in children with tetanus. Spasm is especially evident with slight disturbances in the environment. The generalized extensor spasm noted in tetanus can be distinguished from the generalized muscle spasm of phenothiazine intoxication. The latter does not ordinarily involve the abdominal muscles, but in

---

Decreased Muscle Tone

Malnutrition
General debility, acute illness
Congenital myopathies,
    dystrophies
Postviral and viral myopathies
Neuropathic conditions
Tick paralysis
Cerebral palsies
Lower motor neuron lesions
Cerebellar lesions
Hypothyroidism
Hypopituitarism
Hypoadrenalin
Heavy metal poisons
Mercury poisoning

Toxins, e.g., magnesium,
    botulism
Collagen vascular diseases
Down Syndrome
Ehlers-Danlos syndrome
Prader-Willi syndrome
Peroxisomal disorders
Leukodystrophies

Metabolic
    Carnitine deficiency
    glycogenoses, rickets,
    hypercalcemia, amino acid
    and organic acid
    disorders, potassium
    deficiency

tetanus the abdomen may be boardlike in its rigidity. Generalized flexion or extension spasm may be noted in children with anoxia and is seen in sickle cell crisis, presumably secondary to local muscle anoxia.

Note paresis, weakness, or paralysis. *Paresis* generally refers to weakness of muscle resulting from partial paralysis, and the term *paralysis* is usually reserved for total weakness. These conditions are manifest by the patient's inability to use a muscle after a command or painful stimulus or when the patient tries to use a particular group of muscles and exhibits a lack of motion when attempting certain characteristic movements. Paresis and paralysis may be either spastic or flaccid.

Flaccidity, or flaccid paralysis, refers to the inability of a muscle to maintain its normal tone and position so that it yields readily and without resistance to pressure. The muscles in which it occurs should be noted. Flaccidity usually indicates lower motor neuron lesion and occurs in conditions such as poliomyelitis, amyotonia congenita, myasthenia, tick paralysis, polyneuritis, transverse myelitis, diabetic neuropathy, some drug and heavy metal intoxications, and spinal cord injury. Flaccidity of the lower limbs occurs with thoracic neuroblastoma resulting from extension of the tumor into the spinal canal. Paralysis that comes and goes—periodic paralysis—may be related to potassium deficiency or excess. Paralysis that occurs during expression of a strong emotion such as laughter or anger is termed cataplexy. Diastematomyelia, a spur of bone in the spinal canal, causes progressive flaccid paralysis usually during growth spurts.

The proximal muscles are usually affected first in the muscle dystrophies of adults, whereas primary neurologic disease first affects the distal muscles. This distinction is not as clear in children. Proximal muscle weakness in children likely results from muscle or anterior horn cell disease. Children who rise from the supine position by "climbing" up instead of jumping up (Gower sign) may have proximal muscle weakness of the pelvic muscles. Likewise, they will push themselves up to get out of chairs. Strength in the shoulder girdle can be tested by lifting children under the axillae. If the shoulder muscles are weak, children will slip through the examiner's arms (Foerster sign). Flaccidity may be caused by damage to a small area of the cerebral cortex or to the lateral hemisphere of the cerebellum; these lesions occur rarely in childhood. It is noteworthy that, as in adults with brain injury, paralysis after an upper motor neuron lesion is first flaccid and later spastic. This is also the case in newborns with brain damage; the child may be flaccid for as long as 6 months before spasticity becomes fixed.

In infants, weakness is usually proximal in both myopathic and neuropathic conditions. In children with polyneuritis, the proximal muscles are weaker in the legs and the distal muscles are weaker in the arms. In children with pyramidal lesions, weakness in flexion is greater than that of extension in the legs, but weakness of extension is greater than that of flexion in the arms.

Paresis may also occur with chronic wasting disease, congenital heart disease, rickets, and other forms of malnutrition. Mild paresis may be noted in children with hyperthyroidism. Normally a child can hold the leg extended on command for about 1 minute;

a child with hyperthyroidism can hold it about 10 seconds. Unilateral flaccidity may be noted in children with hemichorea. The leg withdraws on pinprick, distinguishing unilateral flaccidity from true paralysis. Paralysis without other neurologic signs may result from hysteria.

Spasticity refers to a prolonged and steady contraction of the muscle. It is demonstrated by increased resistance to passive movement and gives way suddenly when overcome (clasp-knife rigidity). It is accompanied by increased reflexes and clonus. Note the muscles in which it exists. Spasticity of a limb occurs with any upper motor neuron disease or after a prolonged painful stimulus. Spasticity is also marked in children with the degenerative brain diseases discussed earlier in this section. Spasticity of the extensor muscles of the legs or exaggeration of the postural reflexes with flexor spasticity in the upper extremities is more marked in children with brain damage limited to the motor cortex. However, spasticity of the extensors of both the arms and legs, quadriplegia or tetraplegia, usually indicates more extensive damage in the cortex and the basal ganglia. Spasticity largely of the lower extremities (as in spastic diplegia) is thus usually accompanied by better mental development. Paraplegia (spasticity of the legs with no involvement of the arms) is usually caused by spinal cord disease. Diplegia is paralysis affecting the same parts on both sides of the body; the term is usually applied to paralysis of the lower limbs. The term paraplegia also refers to the lower limbs. Quadriplegia is paralysis of all four limbs but in usage refers to the upper limbs.

Rigidity refers to an absolute inability to flex a joint and is noted in diseases in which there is fusion of the joint. Rigidity of the neck is also noted in children with meningitis and other lesions mentioned in the discussion of the neck. Rigidity of the spine is noted in children with meningitis and other lesions discussed in the section on the spine. Usually the tendon reflexes are absent because of excessive rigidity.

Rigidity with arms flexed, legs extended, and hands fisted in the child in deep coma indicates severe dysfunction of the cerebral cortex (decorticate rigidity). Rigid extension and pronation of the arms and legs are signs of midbrain dysfunction (decerebrate rigidity).

Cogwheel rigidity of the leg muscles, manifested by spasm followed by weakness after flexion, is characteristic of children with myotonia congenita (Thomsen disease). Children with chorea demonstrate a strong handgrip followed by weakness. Those with hyperthyroidism demonstrate good strength in the quadriceps muscles rapidly followed by weakness.

Contractures are observed as fixed deformities of the muscle with limitation of joint motion, frequently accompanied by muscle atrophy. Contractures may occur in any state causing continuous spasm or disease of the muscle.

Muscle *atrophy* is best determined either by noting an obvious decrease in muscle mass or, preferably, by measuring the muscle area and comparing with the opposite side. For example, if you suspect atrophy of the patient's calf muscles on one side, measure the circumference of the calf on both sides at exactly the same distance above the malleoli.

Muscle atrophy may occur after prolonged spasm or disuse from any cause, including immobilization, malnutrition, joint disease, nervous system lesion, and the muscular dystrophies. *Fasciculation* of the muscles is noted as brief repetitive twitches in muscles at rest and is increased by movement of or pressure on the muscle. Fasciculation can be augmented by the administration of neostigmine 1.0 mg and atropine 0.6 mg. They are usually noted in progressive lower motor neuron disease but not myopathic conditions.

Facial *myokymia* (spontaneous undulating waves of contracting muscle fibers spreading across facial muscles) appears most commonly with multiple sclerosis and intramedullary pontine tumors.

Muscle *hypertrophy* is recognized as enlarged musculature with good tone. It is usually compensatory, and other muscles are found to be atrophic. It may result from normal exercise or from constant activity, as in choreoathetosis. In pseudohypertrophy, the muscle appears large because of fatty infiltration; such muscles are weak.

Muscle *percussion* is useful in distinguishing myopathic conditions from lower motor neuron disease. Briskly tap the deltoid, quadriceps, or gastrocnemias. Normally the muscle contracts. Response is usually normal in children with neuropathic conditions but is absent in those with myopathic conditions.

The *superficial reflexes* are the abdominals, the cremasterics, and the skin reflex of the anus, which have previously been discussed.

Obtain the *deep tendon reflexes* of the extremities by briskly tapping the biceps, triceps, patella, and Achilles tendons with the flat of the finger.

Reflex Innervation

Biceps C5–C6
Triceps C6–C8
Patella L2–L4
Achilles L5–S2

Usually a hammer is used to elicit these reflexes in older children. Patients should be relaxed; you should talk casually to them or attempt to catch them unaware to best elicit these reflexes. The muscle to be stimulated should be able to act at maximal mechanical advantage; usually this is a position of about half flexion of the joint involved. These reflexes, though easy to obtain and rarely forgotten, are only a small part of the neurologic examination of the child. Tendon reflexes are stretch reflexes and are elicited by a rapid stretch of the muscle. They are elicited only in the presence of intact sensory nerves from the muscle to the spinal cord, intact nerves in the spinal cord, and intact motor nerves from the cord to the muscle. The knee jerk is usually present at birth and is followed by the achilles and brachial reflexes. The triceps reflex should be present in children at age 6 months. Reflexes may be reinforced by having the child grasp your hand.

Hyperactive deep tendon reflexes indicate upper motor neuron lesion, hyperthyroidism, hypocalcemia, or brainstem tumor and may also occur in areas of muscle spasm, such as early poliomyelitis. Reflexes are hypoactive or absent in the amyotonic or myasthenic muscular dystrophies or lower motor neuron lesions, including polyneuropathy. Patients with cerebellar tumors usually have decreased reflexes. Knee reflexes may be lost early in diphtheria or later in polyneuritis. Decreased reflexes are frequently associated with flaccidity or flaccid paralysis. Flaccidity associated with active reflexes may be seen in children with some forms of brain injury, Down syndrome, malnutrition, and some metabolic disorders. Children with hypothyroidism may exhibit a normal contraction with delayed relaxation of the knee and ankle jerks. Progressive extension of the leg on successive tapping of the patellar tendon (pendular knee jerk), resulting from failure of the leg to return to the resting position, occurs in chorea.

Clonus is a series of forced alternating contractions and partial relaxations of the same muscle and represents an exaggeration of hyperactive deep tendon reflexes. It may be demonstrated as persistence of a rhythmic reflex after a stimulus (such as striking the tendon with a hammer) has been withdrawn; ordinarily, a reflex exhausts itself for a few seconds after it is once obtained. If the clonus occurs with further stimulation, it is said to be *sustained*. If repeated stimulation is necessary it is *unsustained*. It may occur with fatigue or any of the diseases causing hyperactive reflexes.

Clonus of the knee is most easily detected with the lower leg swinging freely over the bed or examining table while the patient is in the sitting position. Elicit the patellar reflex in the usual manner. A hyperactive knee jerk is usually obtained, and clonus exists if the patella or the muscles around the knee joint continue to contract and relax, causing the lower leg to jerk forward and back repeatedly. Clonus of the knee may also occur if the knee is flexed. Grasp the leg above the knee with one hand and the leg below the knee with your other hand; quickly push your lower hand toward your upper hand. You will either feel or see the rapid contractions and relaxations.

Clonus of the ankle is best detected by having the child lie down, with the knee flexed slightly and the ankle resting comfortably with the toes pointing outward and upward. Hold the lower ankle lightly with your left had, and tap the tendon with the second finger of your right hand or the hammer. Feel either the reflex or the clonic movement in the left hand. If clonus is not elicited, place the leg flat on the table with the toes pointing upward; flex the ankle quickly. Feel clonus in the hand causing the flexion.

As a group, increased muscle tone, increased tendon reflexes, clonus, spasticity, rigidity, and abnormal pyramidal tract signs are indications of upper motor neuron lesions, although all these signs may be evident in some metabolic disorders.

Myoclonic jerks are brief involuntary contractures of muscles. Myoclonic seizures, sometimes called *infantile spasms*, usually represent severe CNS disorders and may be an early sign of tuberous sclerosis. Myoclonic jerks during sleep may occur in infancy. If you can induce them by rocking the baby head to toe, they are usually benign.

In infants aged less than 5 months of age, the *Moro* reflex is extremely informative (Table 8-3). Elicit it by startling the patient—either by making a loud noise, dropping and catching the patient, or otherwise surprising the patient. Normally the child reacts as if grasping a tree: the arms first extend, then flex; the hands clench; and the knees and hips flex.

Table 8-3. *Infantile Reflexes*

Reflex	Appearance	Disappearance
Suck	Birth	Through infancy
Root	Birth	3–4 mo
Moro	Birth	3–7 mo
Tonic neck	Birth	3–5 mo
Babinski	Birth	12–24 mo
Stepping	Birth	3–4 mo
Placing	Birth	10–12 mo
Landau	3 mo	12–24 mo
Parachute	7–9 mo	Indefinite

Absence of the Moro reflex in a newborn infant indicates severe CNS injury or deficiency. Persistent Moro reflex after age 7 months has the same significance. Absence of this reflex of one arm indicates fractured humerus, brachial nerve palsy, or recently fractured clavicle. Absence of or irregular Moro reflex of one leg indicates lower spinal injury, myelomeningocele, avulsion of the cord, or dislocated hip. Hyperactive Moro reflex indicates tetany, tetanus, or CNS infection.

A "reverse" Moro reflex consists of extending and externally rotating the arms, with rigidity following the usual stimulus. Such a reflex is seen in children more than 5 days old who have basal ganglia disease, including kernicterus of erythroblastosis fetalis. Such children may have no Moro reflex within the first 5 days of life.

Elicit the *Landau* reflex by supporting the infant horizontally in the prone position. The infant raises the head and arches the back. This is normally elicited from age 3 months to age 1½ years. It represents a combination of labyrinth, neck, and visual reactions; its absence suggests motor weakness, upper motor neuron disease, or mental retardation.

Obtain the *Babinski* reflex by scratching the soles of the infant's feet with something such as a broken, pointed tongue depressor. Normally, the small toes do not move and the great toe moves plantarwise. An abnormal response is one in which the toes fan out and the great toe moves dorsally. The abnormal response is found in most normal children aged less than 18 months. Persistence after age of 2–2½ years indicates pyramidal tract lesion. Sometimes you may find it difficult to decide whether the Babinski reflex is present or absent, since only part of the response will be obtained. In such cases, look for other signs of upper motor neuron lesions before concluding that the response is abnormal. Obtain Oppenheim sign by pressing on the median aspect of the ankle and noting the toes as in the Babinski sign. The significance is the same. Obtain Hoffmann sign by snapping the terminal phalanx of the second finger and noting flexion of the first and third fingers; it too usually indicates a pyramidal tract lesion but is also obtained in children with tetany.

Kernig sign is the inability to extend the leg with the hip flexed and indicates irritation of the meninges, or hamstring spasm. Evaluation in infants aged less than 6 months is difficult.

Obtain Romberg sign by having the patient stand with the heels together. Compare stability with the patient's eyes open, then shut. The patient is normally able to stand without falling. The sign is said to be *positive* if the child leans toward or falls toward one side. It is manifest in children with poor or absent sense of position or the cerebellar ataxias and in cases of vestibular damage and cerebellar tumors.

Foerster symptom is evident in children with generalized hypotonicity. Such children are sometimes called *floppy infants*. Raise the child by the armpits. The legs straighten as the child is raised if the hypotonia results from disease with paralytic weakness such as Werdnig-Hoffmann disease or benign variants of it. If the hypotonia results from atonic spastic diplegia, the knees and hips remain flexed.

Obtain *Trousseau* sign by obstructing blood flow at the patient's wrist or ankle by making a ring around the area with the thumb and index finger or by using the blood pressure cuff. After 3 minutes, carpal or pedal spasm is produced. This sign is present in children with tetany, hyperirritability, or hyperventilation. Obtain the *peroneal* sign by tapping the lateral surface of the patient's fibula just below the head; note dorsiflexion and abduction of the foot. The peroneal sign is also seen in children with diseases of hyperirritability. These signs, in contrast to Chvostek sign described in the section on examination of the face, can be obtained even in a crying child and may be helpful in diagnosing hypocalcemia.

Obtain the *grasp reflex* by placing a small object in contact with the infant's fingers. The infant will grasp the object tightly. This movement is normally present from age 1 to age 3 months. If the movement is absent, brain or local nerve or muscle injury should be suspected. Presence after age 4 months suggests a frontal lobe lesion. With injury to the brachial plexus, the fingers may be constantly maintained (spasticity) in the grasping position or may be flaccid. Infants normally hold the hands as a fist for the first 3 months of life and then begin to hold them open for longer periods. At approximately 6 months of age, the normal infant should begin to take objects with one hand; at approximately 7 months of age, the infant should be able to transfer objects from one hand to the other. After 9 months of age, the infant should grasp with the fingers and appose the fingers with the thumb, and at 10 months of age the infant should develop purposeful release. These responses are delayed in children with mental dysfunction or lesions of the pyramidal tract.

The *thumb position* itself is important in determining neurologic lesions in infancy. In normal infants, the thumb is in a fist in a straight line with the index finger or is freely movable in the palm of the hand. The thumb may be forcibly abducted in the palm of the hand in infants with upper motor neuron lesions.

Evaluate overall developmental motor activity. Delayed appearance of normal motor activity may be caused by brain damage, peripheral motor damage, emotional or mental delay, parental neglect, or to lack of challenge to the infant, prolonged illnesses, or anemia.

A child aged 1 month should be able to support the head for an instant. By 4 months of age, the infant should be able to hold the head up well and roll from the prone to the supine position. At approximately 6 or 7 months of age, the infant begins to sit and is able to roll over completely. At 9 months of age, the infant creeps and, at about 1 year of age, stands with support. The infant walks at about 14 months, runs stiffly at about 18 months, and runs well at about 2 years of age. Children usually cannot skip or throw a ball overhand well until about 4 years of age. For estimation of level of overall developmental motor activity, consult suitable charts or books of growth and development. The importance of the head and chest circumferences, neck and spine mobility, and the status of the fontanels as part of the neurologic examination are discussed in Chapter 4. A convenient table for following the developmental progress of infants has been systematized and should become part of each infant's record (Appendix B).

Sensory changes are difficult to determine in early childhood because of lack of cooperation. Smell and taste, assessed with suitable stimuli, are almost never tested in the young. Blindness and deafness have been discussed previously. Testing of the peripheral nerves in infants is almost entirely limited to the perception of pain. Pain sensation is normal in children with muscle disease and altered in some with neuropathies. Test for peripheral nerve injuries in the limbs by immersing the limbs in warm water for 10 minutes. The skin on the normal side wrinkles; the denervated skin remains smooth. For hand injury, check light touch sensation of the fingertips.

Withdrawal reflexes, which are obtained by applying a mildly painful stimulus and observing unusually rapid withdrawal, usually indicate hyperesthesia and may indicate extensive lesions in the spinal cord. Hyperesthesia is noted early in children with infectious diseases of the CNS, diseases in which intracranial pressure is increased, peritonitis, herpes zoster, and other diseases. Decreased sensation may be noted in children with cord or peripheral nerve lesions, mental deficiency, decreased consciousness, or such states as familial autonomic dysfunction, ectodermal dysplasia, syringomyelia, and congenital indifference to pain. When infants are held erect with the soles of the feet flat on a tabletop, they will take regular alternating steps, exhibiting the *stepping reflex*. Similarly, when prone on a tabletop with the head erect, the infant will make crawling movements. These reflex movements should disappear at about 5 months of age.

In children aged 6 years or older, obtain other sensory responses. Sense of position is described with coordination. Test vibratory sensations with a tuning fork.

Determine stereognosis by asking the child to identify coins or other familiar objects when the eyes are shut. Test *temperature* sensation by asking the patient which end of the reflex hammer feels cooler when the patient's eyes are shut. The rubber end is usually warmer than the metal end. Use cotton to determine sensation to *touch*. Loss of any or all of these means of sensation may be caused by mental delay or decreased states of consciousness. In the absence of these means, abnormal sensory response usually indicates posterior spinal cord root or peripheral nerve lesions, or possibly an emotional disturbance. Increased sensation to touch (hyperesthesia) occurs with chronic illness.

Test the other cranial nerves as a group, proceeding from II to XII. The method of testing response is detailed in the section on examination of the head and neck in Chapter 4.

Table 8-4.   *Some Neurologic Soft Signs*

Physical sign	Concern after age (yr)
Clumsiness in fine motor coordination	
Button 2 buttons	6
Tie shoelaces	7
Alternate left-right, index	
finger-to-nose	7
Finger tapping—each finger with	
thumb, alternating	8
Rapid alternating movements	
of hands (also watch for	
mirror movements)	10
Choreiform movements, tremor	Any age
Gross motor	
Hop	6
Skip	6
Jump	7
Toe walk	7
Heel walk	7
Catch ball, one hand	10
Tandem gait	7
Turning head with eyes	5
Balance on toes	12
Sensory	
Right–left orientation	5
Perceive touch and identify site	6
Graphesthesia recognize numbers traced	8
Recognize objects in hands	5

Other nonneurologic measurements, such as the character of the pulse, respiration, and blood pressure, may again be noted during this assessment as part of the central control of these functions.

Respirations are shallow and irregular with respiratory center involvement. The pulse is weak, rapid, and irregular; the skin is flushed; and the blood pressure is elevated (but may decrease later) with circulatory center involvement. Not only infections and mass lesions cause involvement of the cranial centers; drugs, poisons, acidosis, alkalosis, and water balance may also affect these centers.

A group of signs has been collated as "soft" neurologic signs that may indicate delay in or injury to neurologic development (Table 8-4). These signs are all normal at an early age. Note the child's behavior as the child enters the room and the child's mannerisms and behavior during the interview. Note how the child handles buttons, sleeves, buckles, and zippers. Note ease of onset of frustration and impulsivity.

Finally, note total response of the child, including cooperation, backwardness, lethargy, and reaction to physician and parent. These responses may be recorded in the first statement of your writeup of the child's general appearance. Special characteristics of mental development may also be recorded.

Examination of the Newborn

The baby figure
of the giant mass
Of things to come.

William Shakespeare, Troilus and Cressida, *Act I, Sc. 3*

The infant is a complete individual. The question you want answered is: "Is the infant normal?" Even minor abnormalities should be explained to the mother to allay her fears. In the apparently well infant, a second physical examination should be completed after the infant has adjusted to the new environment, since some physical abnormalities may become apparent after several days of life. However, at the first examination you are restricted to assessing gross physical anomalies. Conduct a more thorough examination 1–4 hours later. You should have an exact idea of what you want to know, proceed with the examination expeditiously, and write it up if even on a check sheet. Keep the baby warm, even preferably unclothed. If the baby is not crying, listen to the chest first. Otherwise, proceed to examine the infant systematically from the head downward. In general, the first examination of the infant consists chiefly of observation of orifices and of masses, bulges, or anomalies, but the method of examination is similar to that already described in older children.

GENERAL

Note the *color* and *breathing* of the baby. If the baby is gray or cyanotic or if the respirations are labored, do not begin the examination until the airway is gently but rapidly cleared, oxygen has been administered, and respiration has become regular. If in clearing the airway of mucus and amniotic fluid a soft feeding catheter with suction is passed first through the infant's nares into the nasopharynx and then down the esophagus to the stomach and no obstruction is met, the diagnoses of choanal atresia, esophageal atresia, and other nasopharyngeal anomalies such as nasal cysts, encephaloceles, and tumors are eliminated. Pass the catheter swiftly and gently without jerking, or laryngospasm may be induced. The tip of the catheter will be seen or felt throughout the left half of the abdominal wall. If the catheter is not palpable, cardiospasm may be present. If the catheter is down but not palpable, hold the hand over the abdomen and blow a quick puff of air through the catheter. The air bubble will be felt. If obstruction is met or the bubble is not felt, consider atresia in either of these areas as a possible cause of the infant's respiratory difficulty. Auscultating over the stomach while blowing air in may be deceptive, since transmitted sounds may be heard even though obstruction is present.

With the catheter in the stomach, aspirate the gastric fluid. Note the amount and quality. Normal amniotic fluid measures 5–25 ml and is cloudy white. Bloody fluid suggests placenta previa. Green fluid suggests meconium-stained amniotic fluid

Table 9-1. *Apgar score*

Criterion[a]	Score		
	0	1	2
Color (appearance)	Blue	Fair	Pink
Heart rate (pulse)	0	100	100–140
Reflex irritability (grimace)	0	Fair	Good
Muscle tone (activity)	Flaccid	Fair or increased	Good
Breathing and cry (respiratory effort)	Apnea, 1–2 gasps	Fair	Prompt, lusty

[a] A score of 8–10 is excellent, 4–7 is guarded, and 0–3 is critical.

from antepartum asphyxia. More than 25 ml fluid suggests gastrointestinal tract obstruction.

If distress persists after the infant's upper airway is cleared, maneuver a laryngoscope of proper size carefully into the vallecula with the left hand, elevating the larynx by pressure with the left fifth finger on the thyroid cartilage; gently push the tongue out of the way with the blade, exposing the larynx.

Shock in an infant is usually caused by heavy sedation of the mother before delivery or intracranial trauma, but it may also result from generalized trauma of delivery, placental bleeding, a ruptured viscus, or hemorrhage in the adrenal area.

Maternal overmedication is a possible diagnosis in a depressed infant who is not meconium stained but who has pallor or cyanosis, a slow, strong, full pulse, and a cord filled with blood. Asphyxia is suggested in a depressed infant who is meconium stained and pale with a slow irregular pulse; soft, distant heart sounds; and an umbilical stump that is limp and contains little blood. Lethargy after the first day is a critical sign of infection, hyperammonemia, and other metabolic disorders.

A helpful evaluation of the baby at 1 minute and at 5 minutes of life is the Apgar score, the baby's first report card. Five criteria are noted, and each is assigned 0, 1, or 2 points (Table 9-1). A score of 8–10 is excellent, one of 4–7 is guarded, and one of 0–3 is critical. Intubate the baby if the score is less than 5. Keep the baby warm.

Gross anomalies such as anencephaly, omphalocele, exstrophy of the bladder, and amelia are immediately obvious; record them in as much detail as possible. Observe the baby for symmetry of head, body, and extremities. Limbs of the term infant are flexed. Failure to move or asymmetrical movement suggests neurologic, muscle, or skeletal injury.

SKIN

Note consistency and hydration of the skin. Normally soon after birth the infant becomes pink and cries lustily. *Cyanosis* in infants is produced by the same biochemical factors that provoke it in older children. Because an infant usually has a higher hemoglobin level than an older child, cyanosis occurs more easily in infants and with less relative oxygen unsaturation than in older children (Chapter 3). Occasionally, ecchymoses will be confused with cyanosis. Pressure on a cyanotic area will blanch the skin temporarily; the ecchymotic area remains blue with pressure. Mongolian spots are usually easily distinguished from cyanosis, especially by their location.

An infant who remains cyanotic may have amniotic fluid, stomach contents, or tumors of the tongue or about the mouth obstructing the airway and causing hypoventilation. Upper airway obstruction may also be caused by choanal atresia, vascular ring; laryngeal web or cyst; hypoplasia of the mandible, or micrognathia, with glossoptosis; tracheomalacia, vocal cord paresis, or injury to the cricothyroid cartilage.

Persistent cyanosis indicates central nervous system (CNS), heart, or lung disease; differentiating between these at an early age is difficult. Cyanosis in an infant with a slow cardiac or respiratory rate, with a bulging fontanel, or with limpness, especially after a rapid delivery (or of a mother who has been heavily sedated), suggests intracranial injury of the baby.

Cyanosis that lessens when the infant cries, especially if the infant is in a high-oxygen atmosphere, suggests the presence of pulmonary disease, such as respiratory distress syndrome, diaphragmatic hernia, pneumonia, asphyxia, or atelectasis. Pulmonary insufficiency is the usual cause of cyanosis in the infant. Increasing inspired oxygen is more likely to increase oxygen saturation in lung disease than in heart disease. Cyanosis that increases when the infant cries suggests cardiac disease. This test of the influence of crying on the depth of cyanosis distinguishes that resulting from solely heart or lung disease. Crying should not be induced in any infant suspected of having brain injury, since the increased intracranial pressure may aggravate intracranial hemorrhage.

Localized cyanosis, which may persist for 24–48 hours, may sometimes be noted in a presenting part. Usually if a normal baby is slightly cyanotic at birth, cyanosis will be less in the hands than in the feet after about 4 hours of age. Equal cyanosis in the hands and feet after 4 hours of age suggests a pathologic cause of the cyanosis.

Peripheral cyanosis (acrocyanosis) is cyanosis of the hands and feet and suggests increased arteriovenous oxygen differences. It is associated with shock, sepsis, and low cardiac output. Central cyanosis involves the mucous membranes and suggests cardiopulmonary disease.

Cyanosis without dyspnea usually occurs with hypoglycemia or methemoglobinemia or if the baby is chilled. Infants at risk for hypoglycemia include those who have diabetic mothers or mothers who use illicit drugs, are small for gestational age, or have asphyxia, infection, metabolic diseases, or hypopituitarism. Cyanosis with little dyspnea may also occur with congenital heart lesions such as hypoplastic right heart, tetralogy of Fallot with severe pulmonary stenosis or atresia, pulmonary stenosis with an intact ventricular septum, and tricuspid anomalies. Cyanosis caused by congenital heart lesions with respiratory distress in the first few days of life requires emergency workup. These findings are present in infants with right-to-left shunts, such as transposition of the great arteries, total anomalous pulmonary venous return, hypoplastic left heart, and some cases of coarctation of the aorta.

Cyanosis resulting from right-to-left shunt without organic heart disease may occur with persistent fetal circulation; persistent elevation of pulmonary vascular resistance maintains patency of the ductus and foramen ovale and may accompany hyperviscosity, atypical respiratory distress syndrome, or hypoglycemia. Cyanosis may occur a few hours after birth in an apparently normal infant with persistent fetal circulation, tricuspid or mitral regurgitation, or other heart lesions. Cyanosis of the upper half of the body occurs with transposition of the great vessels with patent ductus; cyanosis of the lower half of the body occurs with coarctation of the aorta proximal to a patent ductus.

In contrast to pallor in an older child, *pallor* in an infant almost always results from circulatory failure, anoxia, edema, or shock. Only rarely will severe neonatal anemia without shock be manifested by pallor. An infant who remains pallid may have respiratory obstruction, cerebral anoxia, narcosis, cerebral hemorrhage, hypoglycemia, cretinism, or circulatory failure (for example, from adrenal hemorrhage). The pallor of anoxia is usually associated with bradycardia and that of shock with tachycardia. Postmature infants tend to have pallid skins.

A beefy *red* skin may indicate poorly developed vasomotor reflexes, polycythemia, or hypoglycemia in an infant born to a diabetic mother. Occasionally one half of the body may appear red and the other half pale—the *harlequin* color change of the infant. This condition is usually transient and of unknown significance. *Plethora* may also occur as a result of twin–twin or maternal–fetal transfusion and in adrenogenital syndrome. Alternating pink and blue patches may be caused by transient vessel abnormalities or cutis marmorata.

Record evidence of *injuries* secondary to delivery or application of forceps. Scratches, petechiae, and ecchymoses are most frequently caused by injuries incident to delivery. However, *petechiae* and ecchymoses in infants are also caused by sepsis, erythroblastosis fetalis, hemorrhagic disease of the infant, and thrombocytopenic purpura. Rarely, purpuric spots are a result of hemophilia or diseases such as toxoplasmosis, syphilis, and cytomegalic inclusion disease. These spots may occur in infants whose mothers had rubella during the first trimester or who had lupus erythematosus throughout pregnancy. Puncture marks or skin pits may be the result of amniocentesis.

Note any *tumors, hemangiomas, nevi*, and *skin tags*. Telangiectases, or capillary hemangiomas, are frequently found at the back of the neck, the base of the nose, the center of the forehead, on the eyelids (nevus flammeus), or on the mucous membranes where they suggest hereditary hemorrhagic telangiectasia. Vascular nevi may appear over the face or head and may indicate Sturge-Weber disease. Small angiomas may herald angiomas in the retina and brain (Von Hippel-Lindau disease). Pigmented nevi are common birthmarks and may appear any time during the first year of life. Depigmented areas that resemble a leaf and that fluoresce may be an early sign of tuberous sclerosis. Note pigmented lesions of neurofibromatosis, café-au-lait spots, and freckles. Size, shape, color, and degree of protuberance should be recorded. Preauricular skin tags are often associated with severe congenital anomalies.

Scars, usually around the mouth, may indicate congenital syphilis. Examine all skin folds to be certain that the skin moves over the underlying bone. Constricting bands, which are associated with deformity or atrophy beyond the contracture, may be hidden by the folds in the obese infant. They may resemble scars.

The skin of the infant normally feels puffy and edematous. Excess *edema* may be noted in premature infants; in those born of diabetic, prediabetic, or edematous mothers; or in those with hydrops resulting from blood—especially Rh—incompatibility or with intrauterine viral infections. It is noted in children with abnormal salt retention, hypoproteinemia, heart failure, or gonadal dysgenesis.

Note any localized edema in a presenting part that resulted from trauma. Edema limited to the infant's hands and feet may be a sign of gonadal dysgenesis or neonatal tetany. Edema of the genitalia in both sexes is common, especially in infants born by breech delivery. Edema of the anterior abdominal wall suggests perforation of a viscus with peritonitis, appendicitis, or obstructive uropathy. Asymmetric edema occurs with local vascular anomalies, thromboses, or trauma, and Milroy disease, a form of lymphedema.

Edema of the extremities may be caused by heart failure and liver diseases and other causes of hydrops such as blood incompatibility, chorioangioma of the placenta, umbilical or chorionic vein thrombosis, fetal neuroblastoma, cystic adenomatoid malformation of the lung, pulmonary lymphangiectasia, maternal parvovirus infection, Chaga disease, fetal Gaucher disease, and local vascular abnormalities.

Poor *turgor* and excessive wrinkling may indicate dehydration. Dehydration of the infant immediately after birth may indicate poor maternal nutrition, maternal toxemia, defective placenta, or sepsis of the infant. Large babies with good turgor may be born of mothers with diabetes or may be characteristic of cretins.

The *vernix* caseosa, a cheesy white material, is found in the skin folds and the nailbeds. Yellow discoloration of the vernix occurs with intrauterine distress, postmaturity, hemolytic disease of infants and occasionally in infants born by breech delivery.

Desquamation occurs normally in all infants and may be generalized. Marked peeling and cracking of the skin occurs in dysmature infants. Small, hard scales may indicate congenital ichthyosis (known as *collodion* babies).

Redness of the skin with red pinpoint *macules* and *papules* developing in the first days of life are usually transitory rashes caused by irritation, toxicity, or unknown cause. Erythema toxicum may appear within the first 3 days of life and may be indistinguishable from miliaria (heat rash) or varicella. Erythema toxicum has a red base; miliaria does not. Neither involves palms or soles. Redness and tissue necrosis may result from transcutaneous oxygen monitors.

Examine *pustules* carefully. Pinpoint white spots, usually over the bridge of the nose, chin, or cheeks, are most frequently milia caused by retained sebum and are not true pustules. Small pustules that develop after waterdroplike miliaria are a form of miliaria, either miliaria crystallina or miliaria pustulosa. Vesiculopustular lesions, which are shed leaving hyperpigmented macules, are transient neonatal pustular melanosis. Small pustules with a surrounding red area are diagnostic of impetigo neonatorum. If these pustules are associated with *bullae*, pemphigus is present. Pemphigus of the palms and soles of the infant suggests congenital syphilis. Tender, red, indurated areas with sharp borders resulting from streptococcal infection are termed *erysipelas*. In infants, erysipelas may be found near the umbilicus or at the site of a skin injury. Vesiculobullous lesions in an infant may also result from herpes simplex or varicella virus by infection if the mother is infected at the time of delivery. Vesicles may be a sign of incontinentia pigmenti.

Small discrete bullous patches involving the deeper layers of the skin, usually with large hemorrhagic areas, are termed *epidermolysis bullosa*. Small reddish or purple areas of the skin that are hard and movable (fat necrosis) may be caused by trauma during or after delivery but may also indicate hypercalcemia. These areas frequently calcify with hard edges and feel like small saucers or small, loose peas under the skin.

Redness, starting on the face and extending over the entire body and usually appearing in the second week of life—associated with desquamation of large patches of skin—is diagnostic of dermatitis exfoliativa (Ritter disease). In this condition, as in scalded skin or toxic shock syndrome, large patches of epithelium can be removed by stroking the infant's skin (Nikolsky sign). Redness and desquamation in the skin folds represent *intertrigo*, usually caused by sweating and chafing but sometimes caused by fungal or other infections. Erythematous patches occur with neonatal lupus erythematosus.

Jaundice is sometimes difficult to determine in infants. As in older children, examine the skin, the sclerae, the mucous membranes, and the nail beds in natural daylight. Minimal jaundice in a plethoric infant may be more easily discerned by placing a glass slide on the infant's cheek. With slight pressure, the capillary blood and erythema will fade, but the yellowness caused by the jaundice will remain. Jaundice is usually visible in children or adults when the serum bilirubin reaches 2 mg/dL. It may not be visible in infants until the bilirubin level is 5 mg/dL, probably because there is less fat in the subcutaneous tissue in which bilirubin is soluble. Jaundice is usually not seen at birth because light is required to develop the pigment. The yellow-orange color is usually caused by unconjugated bilirubin; the yellow-green color is caused by conjugated bilirubin.

Jaundice in infants apparently progresses from the head to the feet. You can estimate the approximate level of serum bilirubin from the most caudal area of the body that is jaundiced (Table 9–2).

Jaundice appearing at birth or within 12 hours after birth is almost diagnostic of erythroblastosis fetalis. Jaundice after 24 hours is usually physiologic but may also be a result of erythroblastosis secondary to Rh or A-B-O incompatibility, sepsis, congenital syphilis, hemolytic icterus, bile duct obstruction, or viral hepatitis. Physiologic jaundice usually disappears in the full-term infant by the second week but may persist without obvious cause for as long as 4 weeks, especially in some breast-fed

Table 9-2. *Jaundice*

Appearance	Bilirubin level (mg/dL)
Head alone	5–8 mg/dL
Head and chest	6–12 mg/dL
To knees	8–12 mg/dL
Including arms and lower legs	10–18 mg/dL
Including hands and feet	15–20+ mg/dL

infants. Persistent "physiologic" jaundice lasting longer than 4 weeks may be noted in infants with congenital heart disease, especially in heart failure or in cretinism. Sepsis with jaundice is usually caused by staphylococci or *Escherichia coli*. Sepsis without jaundice is usually from streptococci or pneumococci. Lethargy may be associated with jaundice from any cause.

Sweating is rare in infants. It may be present in infants with brain cortex irritation or anomalies or injuries of the sympathetic nervous system or in those whose mothers were morphine addicts or drug abusers.

Congenital skin *anomalies* and deformities are common. A soft swelling, especially of the tongue or over the clavicle that contains fluid and transilluminates, is usually a lymphangioma or cystic hygroma. Midline cysts of the neck may be thyroglossal cysts. Small holes or defects anywhere in the neck and extending up to the ear may be branchial clefts or cysts.

Bluish pigmentation over the sacrum, buttocks, back, or occasionally extensor surfaces is termed *mongolian spots*. It results from pigment cells in the deep layers of the skin, usually disappears in later life when the superficial pigment masks them, and has no clinical significance.

Ectodermal defects of the scalp are common. These usually appear as large, firm, sharply demarcated patches without hair. Look for small holes in the midline of the scalp or anywhere along the spinal column, which may be dermal sinuses. An infected area may be a cause of recurrent meningitis. A defect along this same area (aplasia cutis congenita) with hair over it or the "hair collar" sign, a small nodule with hair encircling it, is a marker of spinal dysraphism (e.g., spina bifida, attachment to dura, or filum terminale). If neural structures protrude through the defect, the mass is termed an *encephalocele* if it is on the head and a *meningomyelocele* if it is over the spine.

Generalized *hardness* of the skin is termed *sclerema*. This condition may result from overcooling the infant and is more likely to occur in debilitated infants, particularly if they have marked alterations in their serum electrolyte levels. Patchy areas of induration of the skin (hidebound skin) is scleroderma and usually does not occur in infants.

NAILS

The infant's nailbeds should be pink. Yellowing of the nail beds has the same significance as yellowing of the vernix. In black infants, increased amounts of melanin are normally found in the nail beds and near the genitalia. Absence or defects of the nails are usually congenital and a sign of either fetal alcohol

syndrome, phenytoin treatment of the mother, or a form of ectodermal dysplasia. The nails may be short in premature infants
and unusually long in postmature infants.

TONE

At birth, the infant is usually limp, but after the first or second
cry, the infant develops good muscle tone. Soon after birth,
infants flex themselves into "positions of comfort," the positions
they occupied in utero. Note areas of flaccidity or spasticity.

Poor muscle *tone* in an infant a few minutes old should be
regarded as a grave sign. In infants who remain limp longer than
a few minutes, suspect anoxia, narcosis, CNS lesions—particularly
edema or hemorrhage—vascular collapse, hypoplastic left heart
complex, hypoglycemia, Down syndrome, and avulsion or subdural hematoma of the cord. Infants with myasthenia gravis may
be limp; they are born of mothers with the disease. However,
many infants who have been limp for longer than several hours
eventually appear to be normal. The cause of prolonged limpness
in such infants is usually not adequately explained. Local loss of
muscle tone may indicate a peripheral nerve lesion. Excess muscle
tone may indicate CNS or metabolic muscular disease.

Seizures may be distinguished from normal tremulousness in
that the convulsing child is usually quiet before the seizure occurs
and the tremulous child is usually active. Soon after birth,
seizures indicate hypoxic ischemic encephalopathy, increased
intracranial pressure from bleeding or infection, anomalies of the
CNS, drug withdrawal, hypoglycemia, or hypocalcemia with
tetany or other metabolic diseases. Tetany is more common in
infants who have low birth weight, diabetic mothers, or asphyxia.
Rarely, omphalitis resulting from *Clostridium tetani* causes
tetanus of an infant with convulsions. Another rare condition,
neonatal nephritis, also causes convulsions.

Muscular *twitching* and hypertonicity have diagnostic significance similar to that of convulsions. However, *tremors* and
twitchings of short duration may be noted, especially if the
infant is cold or startled; these are usually normal and occur in
active infants. Tremors of no pathologic significance cease if you
place a finger in the infant's mouth and let the infant suck. Over
alertness with twitching may result from narcotic withdrawal if
the mother is addicted or, rarely, may indicate hyperthyroidism.
Asymmetric seizures do not help distinguish metabolic from
intracranial causes. Seizures resulting from hypocalcemia or
infection usually begin after the fourth day of life; those caused
by anoxia, birth injury, anomalies, or hypoglycemia begin in the
first 3 days of life. Seizures due to amino acid abnormalities may
present at any time.

Some *facies* are characteristic at this age. For example, Down
syndrome facies can usually be recognized at birth, but cretinism
is usually not detectable until about 6 weeks of age. Mucopolysaccharidoses can be detected only if suspected, since characteristic facies appear after several months. The facies of an infant
with renal agenesis (Potter syndrome) is characterized by low-
set ears, senile appearance, broad nose, and receding chin. Major
facial anomalies may indicate chromosome abnormalities. Note
multiple fractures in children with osteogenesis imperfecta. Disproportion of one side of the body indicates absence or abnormal-

ities of the bone or muscles or congenital hypertrophy. Other representative facies are described in Chapter 3.

HEAD

Note carefully the presence and amount of overriding of the *sutures*. Immediately after the infant's birth, the fontanels may appear to be very small or entirely closed, and the suture lines will be represented by hard ridges. These findings are normal and are considered part of the molding process of a normal vaginal delivery. Within the first day of life, normal intracranial pressure begins to exert its expansive force, and the suture lines and fontanels are felt as depressions in the normal infant. The progress of this expansion is followed during the entire period of infancy but especially during the neonatal period. Failure of normal expansion in the neonatal period may be the earliest sign of microcephaly or craniostenosis. In contrast, rapid enlargement of the fontanels is not a good early sign of developing hydrocephalus; absolute measurements of skull and chest circumference are necessary for this diagnosis. Anencephaly and congenital hydrocephaly are obvious at birth. To detect hydrancephaly, hydrocephalus, or subdural hematoma, *transilluminate* the head of any infant whose head is asymmetric or unusually large or small or who has abnormal neurologic signs.

A tense *fontanel* any time after birth and until the fontanel closes indicates increased intracranial pressure. Except in infants whose intracranial pressure is increased because of crying or coughing, a tense or bulging fontanel is usually a pediatric emergency, suggesting intracranial infection, bleeding, brain tumor, or pseudotumor. Estimate intracranial pressure by raising the infant's head until the fontanel is flat; then measure the vertical distance from the fontanel to the clavicle. Normally, this does not exceed 55 mm in the first few months of life.

A depressed fontanel may be normal or may be an early indication of dehydration. A third fontanel, located between the anterior and posterior fontanels, is a sign of an infant at risk.

Cephalohematoma is frequently not present at birth but appears on the second day of life. The hematoma is soft and fluctuant, and the outline is well defined, with the edge at the bone margin. A cephalohematoma begins to calcify in the first few days of life, and a ridge around the hematoma may be felt for as long as 6 months.

In contrast to cephalohematoma, the *caput* succedaneum is soft but ill defined in outline, pits on pressure, and is not fluctuant. The characteristics represent edema of the scalp, possibly from pressure on the emissary veins. Record the presence of caput, since this may indicate difficult delivery with possible intracranial hemorrhage.

Press the scalp behind and above the ears with the fingers, as if playing the piano, to determine the presence of a ping-pong ball sensation: *craniotabes*. Many normal infants have craniotabes, but if it is present, hydrocephalus and syphilis should also be suspected. The other causes of craniotabes occur later in life (see Chapter 4).

Cranial or facial *asymmetry* is common and is usually caused by intrauterine molding or molding during delivery. Facial or cranial asymmetry may occur in infants with facial palsy, but usually infants with facial nerve injury are not born with asymmetry. Try to assess facial asymmetry as the infant begins to cry. Segments of the facial nerve may be injured and cause confusion; for example, the mentalis nerve and its muscle prevent drawing down the corner of the mouth but spare the nasolabial fold and palpebral fissure. This type of weakness may be permanent. Facial palsy may be hereditary. Central palsy occurs with Möbius syndrome. Facial asymmetry may occur in infants of low birth weight and associated hemihypertrophy (Silver syndrome) and with congenital heart disease in cardiofacial syndrome.

Note presence of *micrognathia* (small mandible). Head retraction may be a sign of a vascular ring causing respiratory obstruction. Chvostek sign is usually positive in normal infants and therefore is of little value in diagnosing neonatal tetany.

EYES

If the infant is crying or keeps the eyes shut, gently rock the head. Usually the infant will open the eyes long enough to allow a thorough neonatal examination.

Note the presence, structure, and equality of the eyes. Edema of the lids may be caused by birth trauma. Real tears may not appear until the infant reaches the second month of life, and the lacrimal ducts may not open until several weeks later. Purulent discharge from the eyes that is present shortly after birth usually signifies ophthalmia neonatorum as a result of gonorrhea or *Chlamydia* infection. Although any discharge from the eyes may begin on the infant's first day of life, chemical irritation usually causes discharge on days 1–3, gonorrhea between days 2 and 5, and inclusion blennorrhea from viral or *Chlamydia* infection on days 4–14.

A mongoloid slant (the lateral upward slope of the eyes with an inner epicanthal fold) or an antimongoloid slant may be variants or may suggest one of the syndromes of mental, physical, or chromosome aberrations. The inner canthal length is normally 1.5–2.5 cm, the outer canthal length is 5.0–7.5 cm, and the interpupillary distances is 3.0–4.5 cm at birth.

At birth, exophthalmos is usually a congenital anomaly, with enlargement of all the structures of the eye (buphthalmos). However, congenital glaucoma is a cause of exophthalmos in infants. An open-eyed stare, common in infants with cerebral palsy, may be confused with exophthalmos.

Enophthalmos is usually associated with ptosis and constricted pupil (Horner syndrome) and indicates damage to the brain or to the cervical spine and brachial plexus root at this age. Constricted *pupil* alone, unilateral dilated fixed pupil, and *nystagmus* or *strabismus* may each be an early sign of brain injury. A searching nystagmus is not uncommon at birth. Later, this type of nystagmus may indicate blindness. An intermittent strabismus is present in nearly all infants at birth but disappears by 6 months of age.

Conjunctival or scleral *hemorrhages* are common and usually have no clinical significance. They may, however, indicate difficult delivery or hemorrhagic disease of the infant. Blood in the anterior chamber (hyphema) is visible as a fluid level when the head is erect and usually indicates more extensive trauma.

Conjunctival edema (chemosis) and discharge may appear a few days after birth and are usually caused by chemicals or eye infections.

Examine the *cornea* for anomalies of the cornea and pupil. Keratitis in an infant may be due to trauma but usually signifies gonorrhea. The corneal reflex should be present at birth but test only if brain or eye damage is suspected. Haziness may indicate cataract or glaucoma. Congenital cataracts may indicate maternal rubella, galactosemia, or disorders of calcium metabolism.

Examine the *retina* and test for a red reflex. Raising the infant's head with one hand is often helpful in getting the infant to open the eyes long enough to visualize the retina. Absence of the red reflex may indicate the presence of lens opacities or retinoblastoma. Retinal hemorrhages usually indicate subdural hematoma or other brain trauma. Chorioretinitis, whitish spots on the retina resulting from congenital toxoplasmosis or cytomegalic inclusion disease, may be found.

The pupil of the infant may be constricted for about 3 weeks or may respond to light at birth by contracting (*pupillary reflex*). Absence of the reflex after 3 weeks suggests that the infant is blind or may have sustained intracranial anoxia or oculomotor nerve damage. The infant's eyes should follow a light. The pupil is normally black to direct light. White pupils indicate opacity in the lens, vitreous, or retina. Detect sixth-nerve paralysis by watching the eye fail to move laterally as you rotate the infant's head in the opposite direction (doll's eye maneuver).

EARS

Note anomalies, position, clefts, tags, and injuries of the external ear. Low-set ears may be associated with renal agenesis or chromosome abnormalities. Because the canals are usually filled at birth with vernix and amniotic debris, you may not visualize the drums; however, they may be visualized at a few days of age. You can estimate deafness at a few days of age by snapping your fingers or making a sharp noise. Normally the eyelids will twitch or a complete Moro reflex will be obtained. In an infant with deafness, there is no such response; suspect congenital deafness, filled aural canals, congenital syphilis, and kernicterus.

NOSE

The nose is usually deformed for a few days after birth, but injury is rare. Test patency of the nasal canals by holding your hand over the baby's mouth and noting the normal passage of air. Since mucus is usually present, a more certain method of testing nasal patency is to pass a soft rubber catheter with suction, as already described. A nonpatent nasal airway at this age is usually caused by choanal atresia or other congenital anomaly. Occasionally, a tumor or encephalocele may be protruding. Nasal discharge may be present normally, and sneezing is common. Thick bloody nasal discharge without sneezing suggests congenital syphilis (snuffles). Sneezing may occur in cretins and in infants whose mothers were receiving reserpine or narcotics.

MOUTH

Note *harelip* and *cleft palate*. Always open the infant's mouth to seek anomalies. Because infants normally have a high arched palate, it may be difficult to visualize the mouth beyond the uvula. Ordinarily, visualization beyond this point is not necessary. Insert a gloved finger to feel for a cleft or submucous cleft, tumors, or thyroid cyst at the base of the tongue. A large tongue usually results from tumor (lymphangioma or hemangioma). The tongue is rarely enlarged at birth in cretins; it is large in infants with Wiedemann-Beckwith syndrome or Pompe disease (glycogen storage disease, type II) and appears large in infants with the Pierre-Robin syndrome with micrognathia.

Infants with brain injury have a protruding adderlike *tongue*. The frenulum of the tongue may be prominent but usually does not restrict motion of the tongue. Obtain the *sucking* reflex (Chapter 8) by placing the tongue blade on the lips, and stimulate the *rooting* reflex by touching the cheek and noting the infant turn and suck; both are normal reflexes present at birth. Absence of these reflexes occurs in brain-injured or debilitated infants and in some normal infants for the first day or two of life.

Teeth may be present at birth. Retention *cysts*, or pearls, are common along the gum margins. Flat white spots that do not rub away (thrush) may be present by 3 or 4 days of life. Small hard *tumors* may be evident in the gingiva, especially in the incisor area (epulis). You may see ulcers, or plaques, on the hard palate after a few days of age (Bednar aphthae) that are usually due to vigorous sucking. Small, white epithelial cysts along both sides of the median raphe of the hard palate are Epstein pearls. *Tonsillar* tissue is not evident in a newborn.

Vomiting is a symptom in older children but may be considered a sign in infants. It is common in the infants aged 1–2 days and may be a result of relaxation of the cardia of the stomach.

Vomiting in Newborns

Sepsis	Malrotation
Cerebral anoxia	Annular pancreas
Increased intracranial pressure	Intestinal atresia
Marked jaundice	Intestinal bands
Adrenal insufficiency	Diverticuli
Diaphragmatic hernia	Duplications
Meconium ileus	Imperforate anus
Peritonitis	Hirschsprung disease
Meningitis	Cretinism
Intestinal obstruction	Metabolic errors
Volvulus	

Vomiting of uncurdled milk or prompt vomiting of anything occurs in infants with esophageal atresia but also occurs in normal infants who have been fed too much or too fast or who have not been properly burped or positioned after feeding. Passage of a catheter with suction, as previously described, helps determine presence of esophageal atresia. Bloody vomitus in an infant most commonly results from ingested blood, but occasionally occurs with hemorrhagic disease of infants or with gastrointestinal ulcers associated with intracranial anoxia or increased pressure. Vomitus with bile suggests an obstruction below the ampulla of Vater or perforation of a viscus; vomitus without bile suggests obstruction above the ampulla. Fecal vomiting usually indicates a low intestinal obstruction. Vomiting also occurs in children with electrolyte disturbances, urinary tract disease, and infections.

Saliva is usually scant until the second or third month of life. In infants, profuse salivation with mucoid secretions may indicate the presence of tracheoesophageal fistula or cystic fibrosis, but frequently it may be caused by tracheal aspiration or irritation.

NECK

The infant's neck is generally not visible when the infant is supine. Bring the neck into full view by placing one hand behind the upper back and allowing the head to fall gently into extension.

Distended neck veins usually signify a mass in the chest or pneumomediastinum. A mass in the lower part of the sternocleidomastoid muscle with limitation of motion of the neck results in torticollis. Small cystic masses in the region of the upper part of the sternocleidomastoid may be branchial cleft cysts. A fractured clavicle may present as a mass in the neck. A midline mass may be a congenital goiter, which is rare, or a thyroglossal duct cyst, which is more common. A soft mass over the clavicle that transilluminates may be a cystic hygroma.

An unusually short, poorly mobile neck may be an indication of the Klippel-Feil syndrome; skin folds from the acromion to the mastoid may indicate gonadal dysgenesis. Excess posterior cervical skin may indicate other chromosome aberrations.

Flex the neck. Resistance is rare but may indicate meningeal irritation. However, lack of resistance does not indicate lack of meningeal irritation, since an infant with meningitis may have a supple neck. Retraction (opisthotonos) may be caused by intracranial injury or infection.

Turn the infant's head from side to side to obtain the tonic neck reflex, which is normally present in infants (Chapter 8). Absence may indicate CNS damage. When the head of a supine infant is turned, the infant's trunk should rotate in the direction of the head movement (the neck-righting reflex). Similarly, if the body of an erect infant is tilted, the infant's head should return to the upright position, a labyrinth response (otolith-righting reflex).

CRY

Note the cry of the infant. The infant should cry lustily at birth. A weak or groaning cry or grunt in expiration usually indicates severe respiratory disturbances. Absence or weakness of cry or constant crying at birth usually indicates brain injury, laryngeal anomaly, or vocal cord paresis. A high-pitched (or cerebral) cry may indicate increased intracranial pressure. Hoarseness or crowing inspirations may indicate laryngeal disease or anomalies. Hoarseness appearing at 2–5 days of age frequently results from laryngospasm caused by hypocalcemia. Hoarseness is usually absent at birth in congenital laryngeal stridor; at birth, the presence of hoarseness requires study.

Hoarseness or Crowing Inspiration

Congenital laryngeal stridor	Laryngeal tumor
Laryngeal nerve paralysis	Thyroglossal tumor
Laryngeal stenosis ·	Mucus plugs

Tracheal stenosis	Laryngeal web
Laryngomalacia	Tracheal web
Tracheomalacia	Congenital heart disease
Vascular ring	Diaphragmatic hernia
Pierre Robin syndrome	Cystic hygroma
Pneumothorax	Abnormal thoracic cage
Bronchogenic cyst	Mediastinal mass
Hypocalcemia	Epiglottic anomaly
Thyroglossal duct cyst	Subglottic anomaly

CHEST

Examine the infant's chest for gross anomalies, tumors, and fractures. The chest is usually almost circular. Depressed sternum may be caused by atelectasis, respiratory distress syndrome, and funnel chest. The xiphisternum protrudes and normally appears broken as a result of the xiphoid's weak attachment with the body of the sternum. Retractions usually indicate interference with air entry. Marked retraction of the chest suggests upper airway, particularly laryngeal, obstruction such as laryngeal stenosis. Immediate direct laryngoscopy is indicated.

Asymmetry of the chest may result from diaphragmatic hernia or paralysis, pneumothorax, emphysema, tension cysts, pleural effusions, pneumonia, and pulmonary agenesis. An asymmetric mass near the neck may be a fractured clavicle. Palpation may reveal congenital absence of a clavicle or of muscle (Poland syndrome).

With a warm hand, palpate for the cardiac impulse. In a normal infant, it is barely palpable. An impulse felt in the subcostal angle or left parasternal area occurs with ventricular enlargement. Increased activity at the apex indicates left ventricular overactivity. Thrills may be felt over the aortic area or suprasternal notch in infants with aortic stenosis, at the second left interspace in infants with pulmonic stenosis, at the second or third left interspace near the sternum in infants with patent ductus, and at the fourth interspace near the sternum in infants with ventricular septal defect.

Enlargement of the *breasts* in either sex caused by maternal hormones is usually evident on day 2 or 3 of life and may persist normally as long as a month. Milky secretions may normally be present. Redness and firmness around the nipple is rare and results from infection—mastitis or abscess. Increased pigmentation of the areola is noted in cases of adrenogenital syndrome. Supernumerary nipples are noted, since they may be associated with internal organ anomalies.

LUNGS

In infant's *respiration* is chiefly abdominal. Decreased abdominal respiration is noted in infants with pulmonary disease, ruptured viscus, peritonitis, or distended abdomen. Thoracic breathing or unequal motion of the chest is noted in those with phrenic nerve paralysis, diaphragmatic hernia, or massive atelectasis. Unequal motion of the chest or deep retraction of the sternum, especially if associated with rapid, gasping, or grunting respiration or flaring nares indicates intrathoracic disease.

Respiratory *rate* is 40–80 breaths per minutes (bpm) at birth. Respiratory movements are irregular in rate and depth in normal infants. Periods of apnea lasting less than 10 seconds may be normal. Weak, irregular, slow, or very rapid rates suggest brain damage. Rates of about 80 bpm suggest pulmonary disease (as described in the section on cyanosis) and transient tachypnea of the infant; rates less than 30 bpm indicate apnea or intracranial injury. Tachypnea without severe dyspnea suggests phrenic nerve paralysis or methemoglobinemia.

Respiratory Distress in Newborns

Transient tachypnea	Central nervous system
Sepsis	Hypothermia
Pneumonia	Hypoglycemia
Pneumothorax	Congenital heart disease
Diaphragmatic hernia	Tracheoesophageal fistula
Myopathies	Neuropathies

Grunting rapid respirations may be the only sign of a very sick infant and may be caused by overwhelming infections anywhere in the body: lung, heart, or brain diseases; anemia; and distended abdomen.

Deep-sighing respirations are noted frequently in infants with acidosis. Increased depth of respiration with cyanotic heart disease results from decreased pulmonary blood flow. Deep respirations also occur with pulmonary hypertension. Decreased depth occurs with heart failure, shock, CNS diseases, and sepsis. Cheyne-Stokes respiration or weak, groaning respiration may be a sign of hypoxia or brain damage in the full-term infant. The *cough reflex* is usually absent in newborns but appears in 1 or 2 days.

During percussion or auscultation of the chest, the infant must lie so that the head and neck are not turned. Increased or decreased areas of dullness or changes in breath sounds may occur simply because of the infant's position.

The chest is resonant shortly after birth. Hyperresonance suggests emphysema but is more often a result of pneumomediastinum, pneumothorax, or diaphragmatic hernia. Decreased resonance indicates improper aeration, usually caused by atelectasis and occasionally by pneumonia, respiratory distress syndrome, or empyema. Atelectasis may represent primary failure of expansion of the lung or may be a result of aspiration of amniotic fluid, food, or other foreign body; thyroid or possibly thymic tumors; other mediastinal masses; diaphragmatic hernia; or chylothorax. Pleural effusion may also be caused by chylothorax or lung disease, including pneumonia.

Auscultation should disclose bronchial breath sounds bilaterally. Air entry should be good, particularly in the midaxillary line. An expiratory grunt suggests difficult air exchange. Rales and rhonchi may be normal for the first 1–4 hours of life due to neonatal atelectasis. Pleuropericardial rubs have no clinical significance. Peristaltic sounds may be heard in the chest with diaphragmatic hernia, although these sounds are frequently transmitted from the abdomen in normal infants. If breath sounds are heard on both sides of the chest and the heart sounds

Table 9-3. *Downes' score*

Criterion	Score		
	0	1	2
Respiratory rate	<60	61–80	>80 or apneic
Cyanosis	0	In air	In 40% O_2
Retractions	0	Mild	Moderate to severe
Grunt	0	With stethoscope	Without stethoscope
Air entry (crying, axilla)	Clear	Delayed	Barely audible

are heard in the usual place, diaphragmatic hernia or pneumothorax is unlikely. Intrinsic lung diseases may cause changes in breath sounds.

A Downes' score to estimate degree of respiratory distress in infants with no pneumothorax, pneumomediastinum, or aspiration can be obtained (Table 9–3). Such a score is useful in indicating oxygen requirements of the baby. A score of 0–3 represents mild distress, a score of 4–6 represents moderate distress, and a score of 7–10 represents severe distress.

Transilluminate with a bright cool light above and below the infant's nipple on each side. Increased transillumination around the sternum indicates pneumomediastinum; illumination elsewhere indicates pneumothorax.

HEART

Percuss to obtain heart *size* or palpate the apical impulse. The apex will usually be found lateral to the midclavicular line and in the third or fourth interspace because of the more horizontal position of the infant's heart. Beware of dextrocardia. A large heart at birth is rare in infants with valvular heart disease, but is seen in children born of diabetic mothers and those with erythroblastosis fetalis, Pompe's disease, or rhabdomyoma of the heart. A few days after birth, however, cardiac enlargement may be caused by heart failure secondary to heart anomalies.

Heart Failure in Newborns

Coarctation of aorta	Septal defects
Patent ductus	Truncus arteriosus
Transposition	Aortic stenosis
Anomalous venous return	Tricuspid atresia
Anomalous coronary arteries	Pulmonary atresia
Endocardial fibroelastosis	Paroxysmal tachycardia
Hypertension	Myocarditis

Enlarged heart with other signs of heart failure may also be a result of peripheral arteriovenous connections, such as cerebral arteriovenous aneurysms. Pulmonary arteriovenous fistulas do not usually cause heart enlargement because pressure on the heart is low. Infants with hypoplastic left or right heart, pulmonary atresia or stenosis, and tricuspid anomalies may also have hearts of normal size.

The heart rate at birth varies from 100 to 180 beats/min and stabilizes shortly after birth at 120–140 beats/min. The *rhythm* is usually regular. Varying rhythm is associated with anoxia, cerebral defects, increased intracranial pressure, and heart block.

Sinus arrhythmia is present in all term and most preterm infants. Absence of arrhythmia is found in infants with respiratory distress syndrome. Tachycardia of more than 170 beats/min after 1 hour may be because of infection, dehydration, anemia, atrial flutter, congestive heart failure, or hyperthyroidism. Bradycardia may be a result of anoxia, CNS disease, long QT, electrolyte abnormalities, medications or heart block, as in neonatal lupus syndrome.

Listen with either the bell or the diaphragm. The first and second *sounds* are almost equal. Splitting of the first sound may be caused by an ejection click from aortic or pulmonic stenosis. Wide splitting of the second sound occurs with atrial septal defect and total anomalous venous return.

Murmurs are noted for loudness, quality, location, and timing, but their significance varies at this age. Murmurs, if present, are usually heard at the left sternal border in the third or fourth interspace or over the base of the heart—almost never at the apex. For the first hour until 15 hours of life, a late systolic or continuous murmur in the pulmonary area presumably originates from a physiologically patent ductus arteriosus. Another innocent murmur is a short, early systolic ejection murmur with or without an early systolic click at the lower left sternal border or pulmonary area, which is loudest at 3 months of age. A third innocent murmur is a short systolic ejection murmur in the axilla and over the back. A soft systolic murmur associated with an ejection click in the pulmonary area may be caused by pulmonary disease. Loud murmurs on the first day of life suggest semilunar valve stenosis or atrioventricular valve incompetence. Loud systolic murmurs appearing between day 3 and day 7 of life suggest ventricular septal defect.

Heart sounds are poorly heard in infants with pneumothorax or pneumomediastinum, cardiac failure, or CNS injury. A single second heart sound may indicate pulmonary atresia or hypoplastic left heart. Clicking or crackling sounds synchronous with the heartbeat suggest mediastinal emphysema.

ABDOMEN

The abdomen is usually prominent in infants. The veins over the abdomen normally are prominent but are distended in infants with peritonitis and pylephlebitis.

Abdominal Distention

Sepsis	Ascites
Low intestinal obstruction	Genitourinary obstruction
Ileal or colon atresia	Peritonitis
Imperforate anus	Ileus

Meconium plug	Meconium ileus
Tracheoesophageal fistula	Tumors
Omphalocele	Large abdominal organs
Pneumoperitoneum	Hirschsprung disease
Gastroschisis	

Visible peristaltic waves indicate intestinal obstruction but may be evident in thin, otherwise normal infants. Peristalsis is normally heard shortly after birth. A silent tympanitic distended tender abdomen suggests peritonitis or necrotizing enterocolitis.

Scaphoid abdomen in infants suggests diaphragmatic hernia or high atresia of the intestinal tract.

Ascites may result from any of the causes of edema (p. 157) and the following:

Ascites

Ruptured viscus	Chyle
Peritonitis	Hepatitis
Necrotizing enterocolitis	Cirrhosis
Portal vein obstruction	Urethral obstruction
Genitourinary anomalies	

The *liver* is normally palpated 2–3 cm below the right costal margin. The *spleen* tip is usually palpable at about 1 week of age. Enlarged liver and spleen are usually palpated or percussed in infants with erythroblastosis fetalis, heart failure, sepsis, trauma to liver or spleen, neuroblastoma, or congenital syphilis. An enlarged liver and an enlarged spleen are also evident in infants born of diabetic mothers and sometimes in those with congenital hemolytic icterus. A liver extending far below the costal margin in the midline, yet not palpable laterally, may result from partial herniation of the left lobe of the liver into the infant's chest with left-sided diaphragmatic hernia.

Left-sided liver is usually associated with situs inversus. Other malrotations are usually not detected by physical examination. The lower half of the right and the tip of the left *kidney* are normally palpated. You cannot diagnose agenesis of the kidney, however, just because you cannot feel the kidney. If the infant is crying, palpating for the kidneys may be facilitated by supporting the infant at a 45-degree angle with one hand at the occiput and neck. Palpate the abdomen with the free hand, and simultaneously flex the neck with the other hand. Abdominal muscles will relax, and the infant usually stops crying. Flexing the knees to the abdomen sometimes also causes enough relaxation. Both kidneys are palpable and are up to 3–5 cm long.

Most flank and intraabdominal *masses* are of renal origin. Enlarged kidneys may be noted in neuroblastoma, Wilms' tumor, polycystic kidneys, or congenital hydronephrosis. A single, enlarged kidney may indicate renal vein thrombosis. The abnormal kidney mass most frequently palpated in the abdomen results from multicystic renal dysplasia, a common form of cystic disease of the neonatal kidney.

The *bladder* is normally percussed or palpated 1–4 cm above the symphysis. Ironically, a greatly distended bladder in the infant is palpated with difficulty because of its very thin wall;

percuss or it will be overlooked. Distended bladder may result from congenital bladderneck or urethral obstruction.

Any other masses palpable in the abdomen must be identified. Tumors, meconium ileus, loculated hemorrhage, mesenteric cysts or other abnormal masses may be found.

Inspect the umbilical *cord.* If the amnion covers the umbilical stump, the condition is termed *amniotic navel;* if the stump is covered by skin, the condition is termed *cutis navel.* Neither has any clinical significance except that the former may be associated with delayed healing and the latter may be mistaken for umbilical hernia. A velamentous cord with insertion near the edge is rare but may signify other anomalies. The umbilical cord normally has two arteries and one vein; examine for this because a single artery may be accompanied by other anomalies, e.g., renal abnormalities or chromosome trisomies. The artery is thick walled; the vein is thin walled.

The cord should be dry and not bleeding. If it is bleeding, the cord must be retied. Redness around the cord after 24 hours, wetness of the stump, or a fetid odor after 3 days usually signifies the presence of omphalitis. A cord that fails to fall off after 2 weeks or a navel that persists in draining after 3 weeks may indicate the presence of a urachal cyst or sinus. Similarly, a child born with a very large and flabby umbilical cord may have a patent urachus. Fecal discharge occurs with a persistent omphalomesenteric duct; this usually indicates Meckel diverticulum. Patent omphalomesenteric duct may result in ileal prolapse, a surgical emergency.

Soft granulation tissue is commonly noted after cord separation. This local condition must be distinguished from the firmer umbilical polyp, which is dark red, has a mucoid discharge, and is related to Meckel diverticulum. Other cysts and tumors of the umbilicus occur rarely.

Ventral *hernias,* with or without diastasis recti, are frequently present at birth and are usually insignificant. Occasionally a child is born with a hernia that pinches off the small bowel. Very large hernias (omphalocele) may be incompatible with life. Omphaloceles are midline, covered by a sac. Gastroschisis is a paramedian defect, usually on the right with no sac. An umbilicus that shifts with respiration (belly-dancer's sign) signals phrenic nerve paralysis.

GENITALIA

Inspect the genitalia. Edema is common, especially in infants born by breech delivery. Pigmentation is usually increased around the genitalia in dark-skinned races but may be a sign of adrenal hyperplasia. Note *femoral pulses, hydrocele,* and *hernia.* The *clitoris* is always large. Carefully inspect the labia. An unusually large clitoris and partial or total *labial fusion* are found in pseudohermaphroditism, usually caused by adrenal hyperplasia. What appears to be a large clitoris may be a small penis. Identify the urethral opening. In female infants the urethral opening is just behind the clitoris.

If the urethral opening is on the ventral surface of the penis, hypospadias exists; if the opening is on the dorsal surface, epispadias exists. Micropenis (a penis less than 2 cm long) may be a sign of other organ anomalies. In male infants, the urethral orifice may ulcerate, especially after circumcision.

The *prepuce* is usually tight in infant males; phimosis does not exist unless the prepuce cannot be pulled back just far enough to allow flow of an adequate urinary stream. Do not retract the prepuce more than is adequate for examination. Small bands and adhesions of the prepuce usually break during the examination. Erection and even priapism may be noted in male infants but usually have no clinical significance.

Palpate the *testes*, whether they are in the canal or scrotum. The scrotum may appear large or bruised, especially after breech delivery. Dark hematoma in the scrotum may indicate rupture of the liver. A deep cleft in the scrotum results in a bifid scrotum, frequently associated with other genitourinary anomalies. A unilateral, dark, swollen, nontender testis may be a sign of testicular infarction.

The vulva is hyperemic. The *labia*, especially the labia minora, are usually large in female infants. The normal labia may be confused with a bifid scrotum. Palpate the labia majora for a small body, which may be a gonad. Adhesions of the labia minora may occur shortly after birth. Because of maternal hormones, vaginal mucoid or bloody *discharge* may occur normally in female infants any time in the first week and may persist as long as 1 month.

Again, use a catheter. Visualize the opening of the hymen. Passing the catheter through the hymenal opening tests for imperforate hymen and vaginal atresia. Polyps or carbuncles of the hymen may be present. These regress spontaneously. The normal uterus may be felt; it is about 2 cm long. Palpate for femoral pulses; absence suggests coarctation of the aorta. Fecal urethral discharges may be present. They indicate rectourethral, rectovaginal, or rectovesical fistulas.

SPINE

Now place the infant in the prone position. Run your hand lightly over the spine. Spina bifida, pilonidal sinus, scoliosis, and the anal dimple are sought. If the *anus* does not appear to be patent, insert the previously used catheter. If the abdomen is distended, perform the rectal examination immediately. Anorectal anomalies, including displacement of the anus, may be associated with sacrococcygeal teratoma. Prominence of one buttock with asymmetric gluteal folds and an abdominal mass indicates an internal sacrococcygeal teratoma.

MECONIUM AND URINE

Although it usually is not considered part of the physical examination, note the passage of meconium and urine. The infant usually voids immediately at or soon after birth. Failure to pass urine by 24 hours of age is highly suggestive of urinary tract obstruction or other urinary tract anomaly and requires further investigation.

Meconium is usually passed during the first 3 days of life. Passage of meconium before birth is diagnostic of fetal intrauterine distress. Failure of passage of meconium by the end of day 2 of life suggests an intestinal tract obstruction, including stenosis or atresia anywhere throughout the length of the intestinal tract, meconium ileus, megacolon, or small left colon syndrome in infants of diabetic mothers.

Passage of small amounts of meconium or passage over a long time suggests a high intestinal or partial intestinal obstruction. Presence of bright red blood in the meconium usually results from ingestion of the mother's blood by the infant, but it may result from hemorrhage somewhere in the intestinal tract—e.g., necrotizing enterocolitis with or without perforation, which constitutes an emergency and which distinction must be determined by suitable laboratory tests.

EXTREMITIES

Place the infant in the supine position. Gently fold the infant into its intrauterine position, encouraging relaxation and maybe even sleep. This position also provides a clue to the range of motion (ROM) normal to that infant. For example, an infant whose hips and knees are drawn to one side in utero will have a greater ROM of the abducted hip than of the adducted hip. Count the fingers. Note polydactyly and syndactyly. Feel for fractures, paralyses, and dislocations of the clavicles and upper extremities. Examine the hips for dysplasia by rotating the thighs with the knees flexed. Soft clicks are common when hips are moved, as described in Chapter 7, and must be distinguished from the sharp click of dislocation. Clicks at the knees are also common.

Multiple fractures with deformity may be a result of osteogenesis imperfecta. Paralysis of the arm may be a result of brachial palsy or fractured humerus. Paralysis of both legs is usually caused by severe trauma or congenital anomaly of the spinal cord. The hands are normally held clenched. The thumb is in the hand like a fist but moves out intermittently. Permanent fisting signifies a cortical thumb resulting from cortical or spinal tract injury.

Test the *grasp* reflex. On pulling the infant upright, the head is normally partially supported. Elbows, hips, and knees generally lack full extension. Response to pain and touch are noted but ordinarily not recorded. Note the tone of the muscle groups. Test passive tonus by moving all the major joints. Paralysis, missed during examination of tone, may be detected. Look for septic arthritis or osteomyelitis in any septic neonate. Examine other nerve and muscle injuries as described for older children.

Palpate the radial *pulses*. Increased right as compared with left radial pulse occurs with supravalvular aortic stenosis or juxtaductal coarctation, Alternate strong and weak pulses (pulsus alternans) are a sign of left ventricular failure. Paradoxical pulse (pulsus paradoxus), in which the pulse changes markedly with respiration, occurs with cardiac tamponade or constrictive pericarditis.

Edema of the extremities may be caused by gonadal agenesis or heart failure and liver diseases and other causes of hydrops such as blood incompatibility, chorioangioma of the placenta, umbilical or chorionic vein thrombosis, fetal neuroblastoma, cystic adenomatoid malformation of the lung, pulmonary lymphangiectasia, maternal parvovirus infections, Chaga disease, fetal Gaucher disease, and local vascular abnormalities.

MEASUREMENTS

Measure and record the head, chest, and abdominal circumferences and the length of the infant. At birth, the head should be at least 0.5 cm larger than the chest or abdomen. If there is any question about developing hydrocephalus, repeat measurements at daily intervals.

With the infant in the prone position, take the temperature by rectum or in the axilla, groin, or other areas if indicated. Temperatures of 33°–34°C (92°–94°F) are common in an infant and rise when the infant is warmed. Low temperatures are also noted after severe birth trauma and severe infection. Aural temperatures are higher than rectal or esophageal temperatures due to brain metabolism. Lower aural temperatures suggest hydranencephaly.

Elevated temperatures are common in an infant who is dehydrated, when brain damage or sepsis occurs, and when the environmental temperature is excessively high. If the temperature elevation at the feet and abdomen is almost the same, the fever is usually caused by the environment; if the temperature of the feet is low and that of the abdomen is high, sepsis is more likely.

NEUROLOGIC STATUS

Finally, the infant's crib is slapped or dropped a few inches and Moro reflex (Chapter 8) is carefully observed. This response, or the lack of it, is valuable in determining CNS status, fractures of the arms and legs, brachial plexus injury, hip or shoulder dysplasia, and recent fracture of the clavicle. An infant with a fractured clavicle may move the arm freely after 24 hours. In infants with Erb palsy the arm hangs limply, with internal rotation at the shoulder and pronation of the lower segment, and does not move as a result of paralysis after brachial plexus injury. In pseudo-Erb palsy, decreased passive as well as active motion indicates an injury to the proximal humeral epiphysis. Moro reflex is absent at birth and improves in infants with cerebral edema. Moro reflex may be present at birth and disappear in infants with cerebral hemorrhage.

Alternatively, Perez sign, another mass reflex, may be obtained. With the baby prone on a hard surface, exert thumb pressure over the spine from the pelvis to the neck. A strong cry will be noted in normal infants, together with flexion of the lower and upper extremities, lordosis of spine, elevation of the pelvis and head, and urination and defecation. Its significance is similar to that of the Moro reflex.

PLACENTA

Before leaving the delivery room, inspect and weigh the *placenta*. Amnion nodosum or vernix granuloma may reflect insufficiency of amniotic fluid, as in Potter syndrome.

Polyhydramnios (excess amniotic fluid) occurs in infants of diabetic, preeclamptic, or anemic mothers; in multiple pregnancies; and in infants with anencephaly, gastrointestinal obstruction, erythroblastosis, tracheoesophageal fistula, and anomalies of the great vessels. *Oligohydramnios* occurs with agenesis of or polycystic kidneys.

Note number of umbilical arteries, cord length, hematomas and thromboses, cord torsion, and inflammation.

EXAMINATION OF LOW-BIRTH-WEIGHT NEWBORNS

A baby is God's opinion that the world should go on.

Carl Sandburg

A low-birth-weight (LBW) infant is one who weighs less than 5.5 pounds (2,500 g) at birth. Infants with LBW may be premature (less than 37 weeks gestational age), with size appropriate for gestational age (AGA), small for gestational age (SGA), or postmature with weight loss from placental insufficiency.

When examining an LBW infant, follow the same principles used in examining a full-term infant. The examination must be even more rapid and less complete and, above all, must be performed gently and tenderly in a warm protected area.

Measurements of the head, chest, abdomen, length, and weight; observation for gross abnormalities; and rapid estimation of air exchange, heart rate, and skin texture usually suffice for the initial examination. Accurate measurements assist in properly estimating gestational age. If a temperature measurement is desired, it should be taken in the axilla; temperatures of premature infants approximate that of the environment. Examination to determine the presence of Moro reflex may be deferred until the infant is more than 1 day old and then performed only by rapping the crib side. Transillumination of the head, if performed, will show large areas of light transmission.

Calculate the *ponderal index*: wt (g) × 100/length (cm³). A ponderal index less than 2.3 g/cm³ is a small index; 2.3–2.7 g/cm³ is normal. A small ponderal index is associated with increased neonatal and sometimes persistent complications.

Normal respiration in a premature infant is irregular and of Cheyne-Stokes type. The average rate varies from 40 to 80 breaths per minute (bpm). A slow rate, rarely a rapid rate, or a regular respiratory rate usually indicates CNS depression. A rapid rate is more frequently a prime indication of respiratory distress syndrome; infection (usually generalized), including omphalitis, meningitis, septicemia, and pneumonia; or atelectasis.

Because the bony thorax is soft, each inspiration is marked by indrawing of the sternum. This collapse of the sternum normally lessens in the first 24 hours and disappears no later than day 4 or 5 of life. Persistence of the indrawing suggests the presence of persistent atelectasis. Marked atelectasis is usually present at birth but diminishes with each breath. Frequently, an infant does well for a few minutes or a few hours and then shows signs of respiratory distress, including marked collapse of the chest wall, rapid respiratory rates, grunting, and cyanosis. Respiratory distress syndrome, foreign material aspiration with secondary atelectasis, pneumothorax, infection (especially with group B streptococci), severe primary atelectasis, pneumomediastinum, and localized emphysema or reopening of the ductus arteriosus with subsequent pulmonary edema should be suspected. Respiratory distress with tachypnea that seems severe but clears in 1–2 days is benign transient tachypnea of the infant. The cough reflex is usually absent in premature infants.

Cyanosis in a premature infant usually disappears within a few minutes of birth. Persistent cyanosis is similar in significance to that in a full-term infant.

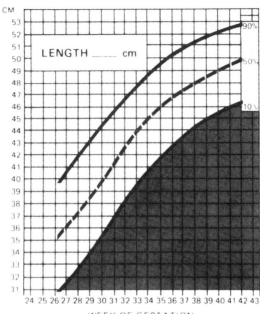

A

WEEK OF GESTATION

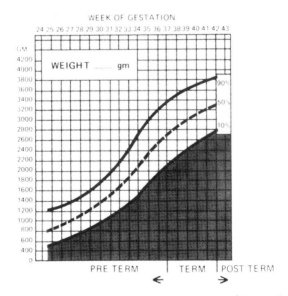

B

Fig. 9-1. Classification of newborns, based on maturity and intrauterine growth. (From Lubchenco LC, Hansman C, Boyd E. *J Pediatr* 1966;37:403 and Battaglia FC, Lubchenco LC. *J Pediatr* 1967;71:159.)

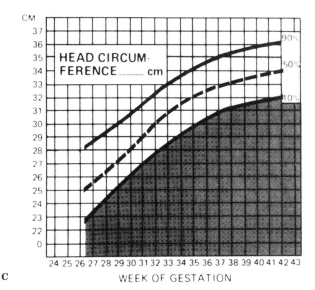

Fig. 9-1. *Continued*

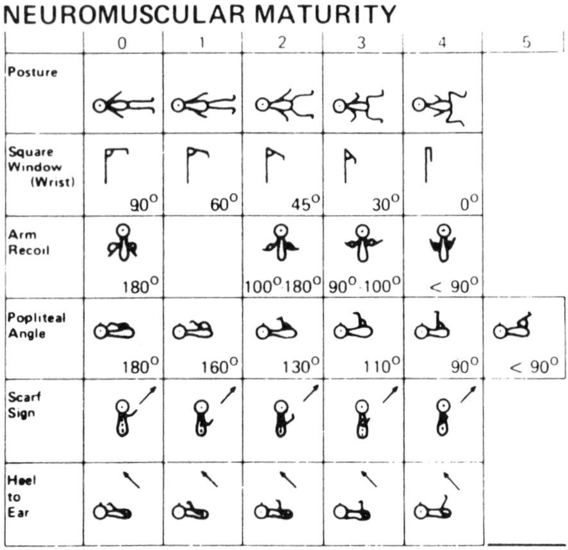

NEUROMUSCULAR MATURITY

	0	1	2	3	4	5
Posture						
Square Window (Wrist)	90°	60°	45°	30°	0°	
Arm Recoil	180°		100°-180°	90°-100°	< 90°	
Popliteal Angle	180°	160°	130°	110°	90°	< 90°
Scarf Sign						
Heel to Ear						

A

PHYSICAL MATURITY

	0	1	2	3	4	5
SKIN	gelatinous red, transparent	smooth pink, visible veins	superficial peeling &/or rash, few veins	cracking pale area, rare veins	parchment, deep cracking, no vessels	leathery, cracked, wrinkled
LANUGO	none	abundant	thinning	bald areas	mostly bald	
PLANTAR CREASES	no crease	faint red marks	anterior transverse crease only	creases ant 2/3	creases cover entire sole	
BREAST	barely percept.	flat areola, no bud	stippled areola, 1–2 mm bud	raised areola, 3–4 mm bud	full areola, 5–10 mm bud	
EAR	pinna flat, stays folded	sl. curved pinna, soft with slow recoil	well-curv. pinna, soft but ready recoil	formed & firm with instant recoil	thick cartilage, ear stiff	
GENITALS Male	scrotum empty, no rugae		testes descending, few rugae	testes down, good rugae	testes pendulous, deep rugae	
GENITALS Female	prominent clitoris & labia minora		majora & minora equally prominent	majora large, minora small	clitoris & minora completely covered	

B

Fig. 9-2.   Add Neuromuscular and Physical to attain Maturity Rating.

Gestation by Dates _____ wks
==

Birth Date _____ Hour _____ am / pm

APGAR _____ 1 min _____ 5 min

MATURITY RATING

Score	Wks
5	26
10	28
15	30
20	32
25	34
30	36
35	38
40	40
45	42
50	44

C

Fig. 9-2. *(Continued)* Newborn maturity rating and classification. (Scoring system from Ballard JL, Khoury JC, Wedig K, Wang L, Eilers-Waisman BL, Lipp R. A simplified assessment of gestational age. *J Pediatr* 1991;119:417–23. Figures adapted from Sweet AY. Classification of the low-birth-weight infant. In: Klaus MH, Fanaroff AA, eds. *Care of the high-risk infant*. Philadelphia: W.B. Saunders, 1977.) **Posture:** Observed with infant quiet and in supine position. Score 0, arms and legs extended; score 1, beginning of flexion of hips and knees, arms extended; score 2, stronger flexion of legs, arms extended; score 3, arms slightly flexed, legs flexed and abducted; score 4, full flexion of arms and legs. **Square Window:** The hand is flexed on the forearm between the thumb and index finger of the examiner. Enough pressure is applied to obtain the fullest flexion possible, and the angle between the hypothenar eminence and the ventral aspect of the forearm is measured and graded according to diagram. (Care is taken not to rotate the infant's wrist while performing this maneuver.) **Ankle Dorsiflexion:** The foot is dorsiflexed onto the anterior aspect of the leg, with the examiner's thumb on the sole of the foot and other fingers behind the leg. Enough pressure is applied to obtain the fullest flexion as possible, and the angle between the dorsum of the foot and the anterior aspect of the leg is measured. **Arm Recoil:** With the infant in the supine position, the forearms are first flexed for 5 seconds, then fully extended by pulling on the hands, and then released. The sign is fully positive if the arms return briskly to full flexion (Score 2). If the arms return to incomplete flexion or the response is sluggish, the score is 1. If they remain extended or if only random movements occur, the score is 0. **Leg Recoil:** With the infant supine, the hips and knees are fully flexed for 5 seconds, then extended by traction on the feet, and released. A maximal response is one of full flexion of the hips and knees (Score 2). A partial flexion scores 1, and minimal or no movement scores 0. **Popliteal Angle:** With the infant supine and the pelvis flat on the examining couch, the thigh is held in the knee-chest position by the examiner's left index finger and thumb supporting the knee. The leg is then extended by gentle pressure from the examiner's right index finger behind the ankle, and the popliteal angle is measured.

SCORING SECTION

	1st Exam=X	2nd Exam=O
Estimating Gest Age by Maturity Rating	_____ Weeks	_____ Weeks

Time of Exam	Date _____
	                    am
	Hour _____ pm
		Date _____
		                    am
		Hour _____ pm

Age at Exam	_____ Hours	_____ Hours

Signature of Examiner	_____
	           M.D.
		_____
		           M.D.

D

Fig. 9-2. *(Continued)* **Heel-to-Ear Maneuver:** With the baby supine, draw the baby's foot as near to the head as it will go without forcing it. Observe the distance between the foot and the head as well as the degree of extension at the knee. Grade according to the diagram. Note that the knee is left free and may draw down alongside the abdomen. **Scarf Sign:** With the baby supine, take the infant's hand and try to place it around the neck and as far posteriorly as possible around the opposite shoulder. Assist this maneuver by lifting the elbow across the body. See how far the elbow will go across and grade according to the illustrations. Score 0, elbow reaches opposite axillary line; score 1, elbow between midline and opposite axillary line; score 2, elbow reaches midline; score 3, elbow will not reach midline. **Head Lag:** With the infant lying supine, grasp the hands (or the arms if the infant is very small) and pull the infant slowly toward the sitting position. Observe the position of the head in relation to the trunk and grade accordingly. In a small infant, the head may initially be supported by one hand. Score 0, complete lag; score 1, partial head control; score 2, able to maintain head in line with body; score 3, brings head anterior to body. **Ventral Suspension:** The infant is suspended in the prone position with the examiner's hand under the infant's chest (one hand for a small infant, two hands for a large infant). Observe the degree of extension of the back and the amount of flexion of the arms and legs. Also note the relation of the head to the trunk. Grade according to the diagrams. If score differs on the two sides, take the mean.

Note the texture of the skin. The skin of premature infants is thin and extremely tender; it is subject to easy bruising, bleeding, and infection and is more subject to injury by temperature changes [which result in hardening (sclerema)] than the skin of full-term infants.

Certain physical signs are characteristic of normal premature AGA infants: a typically round head larger than the chest, prominent eyes, absence of eyebrows and lashes, absence of sweat, purple mottling of the skin (cutis marmorata), extensive hair (lanugo) over much of the body, and soft nails. The neck and extremities are short; the head, hands, and feet are prominent; labia minora are prominent; and the abdomen appears full. Peristalsis is normally visible thorough the thin abdominal wall and is usually not an indication of obstruction. Bloody vomitus in a premature infant may be caused by intracranial hemorrhage, peptic ulcer, necrotizing enterocolitis, or swallowed blood. Meconium may pass during the first 2 weeks of life.

Although premature infants may remain edematous for 4–5 days, they usually remain dehydrated longer than full-term infants. As soon as the edema fluid is absorbed, the skin of the premature infant becomes and remains wrinkled. Jaundice appears and disappears slowly. Many premature infants have umbilical hernias, and the incidence of other hernias, especially inguinal, is higher in premature than in full-term infants. Many premature infants have capillary hemangiomas.

The normal premature infant may seem almost motionless for the first 3 or 4 days after birth. Decreased tone, especially in an SGA infant, suggests hypoglycemia. The child then begins to cry and to make vigorous movements for a few minutes at a time. Early movements usually correspond to the time of disappearance of edema and probably to the onset of hunger. The cry is usually high-pitched in normal premature infants.

The degree of prematurity of an infant can sometimes be estimated by measurements of length, weight, and head circumference (Fig. 9-1) and by their comparison with those of a term infant. Attempt to estimate gestational age as accurately as possible. Infants of LBW may be of decreased gestational age, or the LBW may be caused by various maternal, placental, or fetal factors. The prognoses of these two groups differ. A scoring system has been helpful in making more precise determination of gestational age (Fig. 9-2). Because the incidence of severe congenital anomalies is higher in premature than in full-term infants, such anomalies must also be sought.

Appendix A: Record of Physical Examination

Temp _____ Pulse _____ Resp _____ BP _____
Age _____ Sex _____ Ht _____ Wt _____
Head circ _____ Chest circ _____
Skin folds_____

General appearance: Ill or well, distressed, alert, cooperative, body build. Reaction to parents. Facies. Characteristic position, movements, nutrition, development. Speech.

Skin: Color, pigmentation, cyanosis. Veins, arteries, thrombophlebitis. Jaundice, carotenemia. Pallor. Eruptions. Petechiae. Ecchymosis. Hives. Dermatographia. Tache cerebrale. Subcutaneous nodules. Xanthomas. Texture. Scaling, striae, scars, sweat, subcutaneous tissue, emphysema. Turgor, edema.

Nails: Cyanosis, pallor, pulsations, pitting, hemorrhages.

Hair (body): Distribution, color.

Lymph nodes: Occipital, postauricular, cervical, parotid, submaxillary, sublingual, axillary, epitrochlear, inguinal. Size, mobility, tenderness, heat.

Head: Position, hair, shape, sutures, fontanels. Circumference. Microcephaly, hydrocephaly. Craniotabes, Macewen's sign. Percussion, sinuses. Auscultation, bruit, veins.

Face: Shape. Facial paralysis, trigeminal paralysis. Swelling; parotid, submaxillary, sublingual glands. Facial appearance, hypertelorism, twitching, Chvostek's sign.

Eyes: Vision, visual fields. Blinking. Scleras, exophthalmos, enophthalmos. Strabismus. Ocular movement. Nystagmus. Ptosis, eyelids. Conjunctivae, pingueculae, pterygium, sties, chalazion, blepharitis. Cornea, discharge. Pupils, accommodation, iris. Retina, red reflex, fundus, vessels, hemorrhage, chorioretinitis, disc, macula. Corneal reflex.

Ears: Anomaly, position. Discharge. Tenderness. Canals. Drums, redness, light reflex, landmarks, bulging, perforation, mobility. Mastoids, nodes. Hearing. Vestibular function.

Nose: Shape. Alae nasi, flaring. Mucosa, secretions, bleeding, airway. Septum. Polyps, tumor, encephalocele. Sinuses.

Lips: Paralysis, cleft, fissures, vesicles, color, edema.

Mouth, Throat: Odors, trismus. Circumoral pallor. Teeth, number, edges, occlusion, caries, formation, color. Salivation.

Gums: Infection, discoloration, bleeding, cysts. Buccal mucosa, thrush, veins.

Tongue: Coating, moisture, tremor, papillae, color, geographic, furrows, scars, size, tongue-tie, cysts, paralysis.

Palate: Color, bleeding, cleft, perforation, arch. Epiglottis. Uvula, soft palate. Posterior pharynx. Tonsils, infections, size. Postnasal drip. Koplik's spots, eruptions, ulcers.

Larynx: Voice. Laryngoscopy. Speech.

Neck: Size, anomalies, webbing, edema, nodes, masses. Sternocleidomastoids. Trachea. Thyroid. Vessels. Motion, opisthotonos, Brudzinski's sign, tonic neck reflex. Head drop. Tilting. Nodding.

Chest: Inspection, shape, circumference, rosary, Harrison's groove, flaring, angle, expansion; abdominal, thoracic, intercostal motion, retraction, symmetry, scapulae.

Breasts: Observation, development, symmetry, redness, heat, tenderness, masses. Tanner stage.

Lungs: Respiration. Type, Cheyne-Stokes. Rate, Tachypnea, slow, apnea, Biot's. Depth, hyperpnea. Dyspnea, exercise tolerance. Cough, hemoptysis, sputum, cough reflex. Palpation, masses, tenderness, thud, fremitus; interspaces, retraction, paralysis; pulsations, friction rubs, nodes. Percussion, dullness, scapulae, diaphragm, liver, heart, mediastinum, hyperresonance. Auscultation, sounds, rales, rub, slap, rhonchi, wheezes, vocal resonance, peristalsis.

Heart: Inspection, bulging, impulse; distress, cyanosis, edema, clubbing, pulsations, vessels, femoral pulse, blood pressure. Pulse rate, tachycardia, pulsus alternans, bradycardia, water-hammer, thready, dicrotic, pulsus paradoxus. Arrhythmia, premature beats, extrasystoles, rhythm, fibrillation. Palpation, size, apex impulse, tenderness, thrill. Percussion. Auscultation, sounds, quality, split, third sound, gallop, tic-tac, friction rub, venous hum, murmurs. Failure.

Abdomen: Inspection, shape, distention, transillumination, respiration. Umbilicus, diastasis, veins. Peristalsis. Gastric waves. Auscultation. Percussion, fluid, masses. Palpation, superficial, tense, tenderness, rebound; spleen, liver, masses. Deep palpation, ballottement, bladder, kidneys, reflexes. Femoral pulses, hydration, consistency.

Genitalia: Discharge, foreign body, caruncle, prolapse. Labia, adhesions, vagina, clitoris. Penis, hypospadias, epispadias, phimosis. Scrotum, testes, hydrocele, hernia. Cremasteric reflex, nodes. Tanner stage.

Anus and rectum: Buttocks. Fistula. Fissure. Prolapse. Polyps. Hemorrhoids. Diaper rash. Rectum, fistula, megacolon, masses, prostate, uterus, tenderness. Sensation.

Extremities: Anomalies, length, clubbing, pain, tenderness, temperature, gangrene, swelling, deformities, shape. Feet. Gait, stance, balance, limp, ataxia.

Spine: Hair, dimples, masses, spina bifida, tenderness, mobility. Opisthotonos, scapulae. Posture, lordosis, kyphosis, scoliosis.

Joints: Heat, tenderness, swelling, effusion, redness, motion. Hip dysplasia.

Muscles: Development, tone, tenderness, spasm, paralysis, rigidity, contractures, atrophy.

Nervous system: General impression, abilities, responsiveness, position, spontaneous movements, play activity, development. State of consciousness, irritability, convulsive states. Gait, stance, limp, ataxia. Coordination. Tremors, twitching, choreiform movement, athetosis, associated movements. Rigidity, paresis, paralysis, spasticity, flaccidity. Reflexes, superficial, tendon, clonus. Moro tonic neck. Babinski, Oppenheim Hoffmann, Kernig, Romberg, Foerster, Trousseau, peroneal, Chvostek's grasp. Thumb position. Neck and spine mobility, fontanels. Sensation, blind, deaf, withdrawal reflex, hyperesthesia, hypesthesia, position, vibration, temperature, touch. Astereognosis. Cranial nerves I–XII.

Appendix B: The Denver II Revision and Restandardization of the Denver Developmental Screening test

Because services for handicapped children have markedly expanded since the Denver Developmental Screening Test (DDST) first appeared in 1967, the test has undergone a major revision and restandardization. A pool of 350 potential items was developed through a review of existing items and the creation of additional ones. Criteria for the administration and interpretation of each item were developed. The items were standardized on two samples. The first sample, Denver County (N = 1,039), was subdivided into three ethnic groups, each of which was further divided on the basis of maternal education. Each of these was again divided into 10 age categories; the second sample, the Colorado non-Denver sample (N = 1,057), was subdivided into three residence categories (rural, suburban, urban), and each was further subdivided on the basis of maternal education and age of children, similar to the Denver County sample.

Each item was examined by regression analysis to determine the age at which 25, 50, 75, and 90% of children in each subject/group could perform the item. A goodness-of-fit test was applied to the data to determine the accuracy of the curves. Tester–observer and test–retest reliability was determined for each item.

The final selection of 125 items was made on the basis of eight criteria. Changes in times were an increase of 85% in language items, the addition of two items on speech intelligibility, and a decrease of 22% in the number of report items.

The 125 items are displayed on a test form that has an age scale corresponding to the American Academy of Pediatrics (AAP) recommended health maintenance visits. The test form also includes a behavior rating scale (Fig. B-1).

Currently, the Denver II screening manual, test form, and proficiency test are being used in diverse parts of the United States. For interpretation purposes, the *Denver II Technical Manual* contains norms of subgroups having significantly different ages at which 90% of children pass the item as compared with the group norms that are presented on the test form.

Detailed administration and scoring instructions are given in the *Denver II Screening Manual*, which must be used to ensure accuracy in administration of the test. These materials are available from DDM, Inc., P.O. Box 6919, Denver, CO 80206-0919.

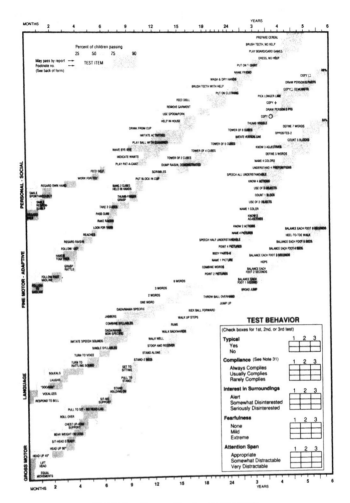

Fig. B-1. Denver Developmental Scale.

DIRECTIONS FOR ADMINISTRATION

1. Try to get child to smile by smiling, talking or waving. Do not touch him/her.
2. Child must stare at hand several seconds.
3. Parent may help guide toothbrush and put toothpaste on brush.
4. Child does not have to be able to tie shoes or button/zip in the back.
5. Move yarn slowly in an arc from one side to the other, about 8" above child's face.
6. Pass if child grasps rattle when it is touched to the backs or tips of fingers.
7. Pass if child tries to see where yarn went. Yarn should be dropped quickly from sight from tester's hand without arm movement.
8. Child must transfer cube from hand to hand without help of body, mouth, or table.
9. Pass if child picks up raisin with any part of thumb and finger.
10. Line can vary only 30 degrees or less from tester's line. ⎍
11. Make a fist with thumb pointing upward and wiggle only the thumb. Pass if child imitates and does not move any fingers other than the thumb.

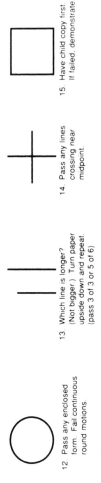

12. Pass any enclosed form. Fail continuous round motions.

13. Which line is longer? (Not bigger.) Turn paper upside down and repeat (pass 3 of 3 or 5 of 6)

14. Pass any lines crossing near midpoint.

15. Have child copy first. If failed, demonstrate.

16. When giving items 12, 14, and 15, do not name the forms. Do not demonstrate 12 and 14.
17. When scoring, each pair (2 arms, 2 legs, etc.) counts as one part.

17. Place one cube in cup and shake gently near child's ear, but out of sight. Repeat for other ear.

Fig. B-1.   Continued

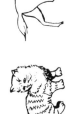
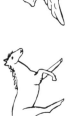
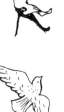
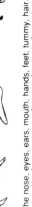

18. Point to picture and have child name it. (No credit is given for sounds only.) If less than 4 pictures are named correctly, have child point to picture as each is named by tester.

19. Using doll, tell child: Show me the nose, eyes, ears, mouth, hands, feet, tummy, hair. Pass 6 of 8.
20. Using pictures, ask child: Which one flies?... says meow?... talks?... barks?... gallops? Pass 2 of 5, 4 of 5.
21. Ask child: What do you do when you are cold?... tired?... hungry? Pass 2 of 3, 3 of 3.
22. Ask child: What do you do with a cup? What is a chair used for? What is a pencil used for? Action words must be included in answers.
23. Pass if child correctly places and says how many blocks are on paper. (1, 5).
24. Tell child: Put block **on table, under table, in front of** me, **behind** me. Pass 4 of 4. (Do not help child by pointing, moving head or eyes.)
25. Ask child: What is a ball?... lake?... desk?... house?... banana?... curtain?... ceiling? Pass if defined in terms of use, shape, what it is made of, or general category (such as banana is fruit, not just yellow). Pass 5 of 8, 7 of 8.
26. Ask child: If a horse is big, a mouse is ___? If fire is hot, ice is ___? If the sun shines during the day, the moon shines during the ___? Pass 2 of 3.
27. Child may use wall or rail only, not person. May not crawl.
28. Child must throw ball overhand 3 feet to within arm's reach of tester.
29. Child must perform standing broad jump over width of test sheet (8 1/2 inches).
30. Tell child to walk forward, heel within 1 inch of toe. Tester may demonstrate.
31. Child must walk 4 consecutive steps.
32. In the second year, half of normal children are non-compliant.

OBSERVATIONS:

Fig. B-1. Continued

Appendix C: Physical Growth and the Early Language Milestone Scale

The charts of head circumference in boys and girls from age 1 month to age 18 years are shown in Fig. C-1. Figures C-2–7 show physical growth percentiles for boy and girls from birth to 18 years of age. Figure 8 and the following text* present the Early Language Milestone (ELM) Scale.

The ELM Scale is a tool for assessing language development from birth to 36 months of age and intelligibility of speech from birth to 48 months of age. Language is assessed independently in three areas: auditory expressive, auditory receptive, and visual. Auditory expressive development is subdivided into content (such as cooing, babbling, single words, two-word phrases) and intelligibility (clarity of speech). Auditory receptive development includes prelinguistic auditory behaviors (orienting to voice or bell), plus comprehension of progressively more complex verbal commands. Visual language includes prelinguistic behaviors (visual tracking and response to facial expressions) and symbolic features such as pointing to desired objects. Item V10 (index finger pointing) characterizes an ability that emerges at the same age as that described by item AE 9 (first word) and implies the same degree of linguistic competence. The ELM Scale may be scored on a pass/fail basis or may be converted to point scores and percentile values for auditory expressive, auditory receptive, visual, and global language function.

I. General Instructions

a) Draw vertical line down entire page at child's chronologic age (CA).

b) Work *backward* from CA, until three consecutive items in each Division (AE, AR, V) are passed (=Basal Level).

c) If child achieves Basal without failing any items already attained by more than 90% of children, *stop*. ELM screen is passed.

d) If one or more items that have already been attained by more than 90% of children are failed, work *forward* from CA until three consecutive items in that Division are failed. (Exception: Child is permitted to fail *one* of the following without penalty: V3–V6). The 50% value of the highest item passed in each Division is the Ceiling Level.

If Ceiling Level ≥ CA→ELM screen is passed.
If Ceiling Level < CA→ELM screen is failed.

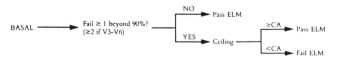

* (From Coplan J: *The Early Language Milestone Scale*. Austin, TX: PRO-ED, 1987.)

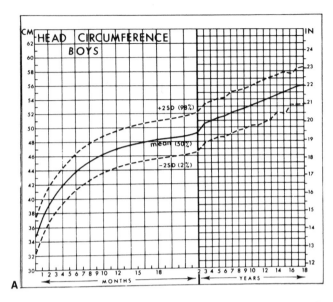

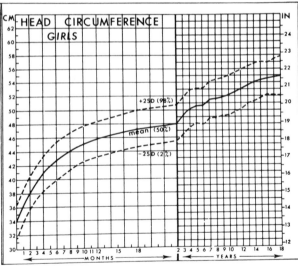

Fig. C-1.   Head circumference in boys and girls from 1 month to 18 years of age.

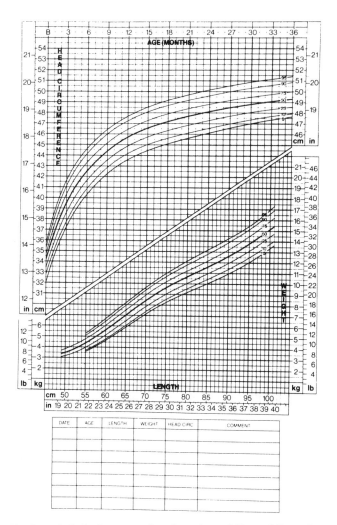

Fig. C-2.   Girls: Birth to 36 months—physical growth National Center for Health Statistics (NCHS) percentiles. (Modified from Hamill PV, Drizd TA, Johnson CL, Reed RB, Roche AF, Moore WM: Physical growth: National Center for Health Statistics percentiles. *Am J Clin Nutr* 1979;32:607–29. Data from the Fels Research Institute, Wright State University School of Medicine, Yellow Springs, OH. Courtesy Ross Laboratories, Columbus, OH.)

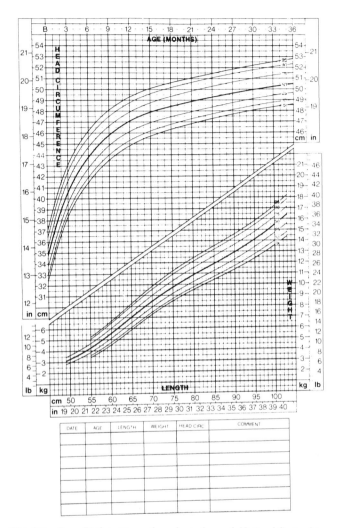

Fig. C-3. Boys: Birth to 36 months—physical growth National Center for Health Statistics (NCHS) percentiles. (Modified from Hamill PV, Drizd TA, Johnson CL, Reed RB, Roche AF, Moore WM: Physical growth: National Center for Health Statistics percentiles. *Am J Clin Nutr* 1979;32:607–29. Data from the Fels Research Institute, Wright State University School of Medicine, Yellow Springs, OH.)

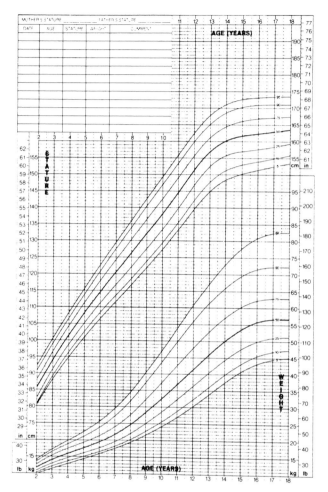

Fig. C-4. Girls: 2–18 years—physical growth National Center for Health Statistics (NCHS) percentiles. (Modified from Hamill PV, Drizd TA, Johnson CL, Reed RB, Roche AF, Moore WM: Physical growth: National Center for Health Statistics percentiles, *Am J Clin Nutr* 1979;32:607–629. Data from the National Center for Health Statistics [NCHS], Hyattsville, MD.)

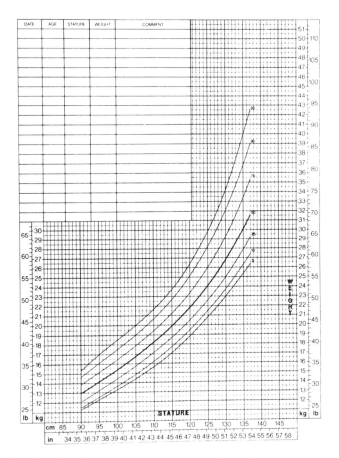

Fig. C-5. Girls: Prepubescent—physical growth National Center for Health Statistics (NCHS) percentiles. (Modified from Hamill PV, Drizd TA, Johnson CL, Reed RB, Roche AF, Moore WM: Physical growth: National Center for Health Statistics percentiles. *Am J Clin Nutr* 1979;32:607–29. Data from the National Center for Health Statistics, Hyattsville, MD.)

II. Auditory Expressive (AE)

a. Content

AE1:   Prolonged musical vowel sounds in a sing-song fashion (ooo, aaa, etc.), *not* just grunts or squeaks.

AE2 H: "Does baby watch speaker's face and appear to listen intently, then vocalize when the speaker is quiet? Can you 'have a conversation' with your baby?"

AE4 H: Blow bubbles or "bronx cheer"?

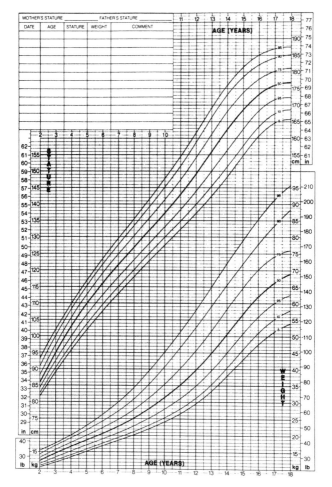

Fig. C-6.   Boys: 2 to 18 years—physical growth National Center for Health Statistics (NCHS) percentiles. (Modified from Hamill PV, Drizd TA, Johnson CL, Reed RB, Roche AF, Moore WM: Physical growth: National Center for Health Statistics percentiles. *Am J Clin Nutr* 1979;32:607–29. Data from the National Center for Health Statistics, Hyattsville, MD.)

AE5 H: Isolated sounds such as ba, da, ga, goo, etc.

AE6 H: Repetitive string of sounds: "baba-baba" or "lalalalala," etc.

AE7 H: Says "mama" or "dada," but uses them at other times besides just labeling parents.

AE8 H: Child *spontaneously, consistently,* and *correctly* uses "mama" or "dada," *just* to label the *appropriate* parent.

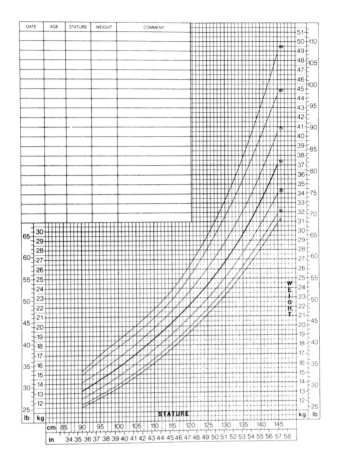

Fig. C-7. Boys: Prepubescent—physical growth National Center for Health Statistics (NCHS) percentiles. (Modified from Hamill PV, Drizd TA, Johnson CL, Reed RB, Roche AF, Moore WM: Physical growth: National Center for Health Statistics percentiles. *Am J Clin Nutr* 1979;32:607–29. Data from the National Center for Health Statistics, Hyattsville, MD.)

AE9, AE10 H: Child *spontaneously, consistently, and correctly* uses words. Do not count "mama," "dada," or the names of other family members or pets. *Do* list the particular words.

AE11 H: Uses single words to tell you demands. "Milk!" "Cookie!" "More!" etc. Pass = two or more wants. List specific words.

AE12 H: *Spontaneous, novel* two-word combinations ("Want cookie," "No bed," "See daddy," etc.) *Not* rotely learned

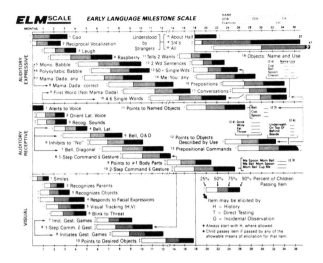

Fig. C-8.   The Early Language Milestone Scale. The horizontal axis is the age in months.

phrases that have been specifically taught to the child or combinations that are really single thoughts (e.g., "hot dog").

AE14 H: Child uses "me" or "you" but may reverse them ("you want cookie" instead of "me want cookie," etc.)

AE17 H: "Can child put two or three sentences together to hold brief conversations?"

AE18 T: Put out cup, ball, crayon, and spoon. Pick up cup and say, "What is this? What do we do with it? What is it for?" Child must *name* the object and give its use. Pass = "drink with," etc., *not* "milk" or "juice." Ball: Pass = "throw," "play with," etc. Spoon: Pass = "Eat" or "Eat with," etc., *not* "Food," "Lunch." Crayon: Pass = "Write (with)," "Color (with)," etc. Pass item if child gives *name and use* for two objects.

b. Intelligibility
AE15, AE19, AE20: "How clear are the words your child makes? That is, how much of your child's speech can a stranger understand?"

——Less than half
——About half (AE15)   Pick
——Three quarters (AE19)   one
——All or almost all (AE20)   (H,O)

To Score:
If "less than half": Fail all three items in cluster
If "about half": Pass AE15 only
If "three quarters": Pass AE19 and AE15
If "all or almost all": Pass all three items in cluster

III. Auditory Receptive (AR)

AR1 H, T: Any behavioral change in response to noise (eye blink, startle, change in movements or respiration, etc.)

AR2 H, T: What does baby do when mother starts talking while out of baby's line of sight? Pass if any shift of head or eyes to voice.

AR3 H: Does baby seem to respond in a specific way to certain sounds (becomes excited at hearing parents' voices, etc.)?

AR4 T: Sit facing baby, with baby in mother's lap. Extend both arms so that your hands are behind baby's field of vision and at the level of baby's waist. Ring a 2-inch diameter bell, first with one hand, then the other. Repeat × 2 or × 3 if necessary. Pass if baby turns head to the side at least once.

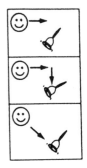

AR5 T: See note for AR4. Pass if baby turns head first to the side, then down to localize bell at least once. (Automatically passes AR4.)

AR6 H: Does baby understand the command "No" (even though baby may not always obey)?

AR6 T: Test by commanding, "(*Baby's name*), no!" while baby is playing with any test object. Pass if baby temporarily inhibits actions.

AR7 T: See note for AR4. Pass if baby turns directly down on diagonal to localize bell at least once. (Automatically passes AR5 and AR4.)

AR8 H: Will your baby follow any verbal commands *without* you indicating by gestures what the action is ("Stop," "Come here," "Give me," etc.)?

AR8 T: Wait until baby is playing with any test object, then say, "(*Baby's name*), give it to me." Pass if baby extends object to you, even if baby seems to change mind and takes the object back. May repeat command × 1 or × 2. If the test failed, repeat the command, but this time hold out your hand for the object. If baby responds, then pass item V8 (one step command with gesture).

AR9 H: Does your child point to at least one body part on command?

AR9 T: Have mother command baby, "Show me your . . ." or "Where's your . . ." without pointing to the desired part herself.

AR10 H: Can child do two things in a row if asked? For example, "First go get your shoes, then sit down."

AR10 T: Set out ball, cup, sand spoon and say, "(*Child's name*), give me the spoon, then give the ball to mommy." Use slow, steady voice but do *not* break command into two separate sentences. If no response, *then* give each half of command separately to see if child understands separate components. If child succeeds on at least half of command, then give each of the following: "(*Child's name*), give me the ball and give mommy the spoon." May repeat once, but do not break into two commands. Then, "Give mommy the ball, then give the cup to me." Pass if at least two two-step commands are executed correctly. (Note: Child is credited even if the order of execution of a command is reversed.)

AR11 H: Place a cup, ball, and spoon on the table. Command child, "Show me/where is/give me the . . . cup/ball/spoon. (If command is "Give me," be sure to replace each object before asking about the next object.) Pass = two items correctly identified.

AR12 T: Put cup, ball, spoon, and crayon on table and give command, "Show me/where is/give me . . . the one we drink with/eat with/draw (color, write) with/throw (play with)." If the command "Give me" is used, be sure to replace each object before asking about the next object. Pass = two or more objects correctly identified.

AR13: Put out cup (upside down) and a 1-inch red cube. Command the child, "Put the block underneath the cup." Repeat × 1 or × 2 if necessary. If no attempt or if incorrect response, then demonstrate correct response, saying, "See now the block is *underneath* the cup." Remove the block and hand it to the child. Then give command, "Put the block *on top* of the cup": If child makes no response, then repeat command × 1 but do *not* demonstrate. Then command, "Put the block *behind* the cup," then "Put the block *beside* the cup." Pass = two or more commands correctly executed (*before* demonstration by examiner, if "underneath" is scored).

IV. Visual

V1 H: "Does your baby smile for you? Not just a gas bubble or a burp, but a real smile?"

V1 T: Have mother attempt to elicit smile by any means.

V2 H: "Does your baby seem to recognize you, reacting differently to you than to the sight of other people? For example, does your baby smile more quickly for you than for other people?"

V3 H: "Does your baby seem to recognize any common objects by sight? For example (if bottle or spoon fed), what happens when bottle or spoon is brought into view but *before* it touches baby's lips?" Pass if baby gets visibly excited or opens mouth in anticipation of feeding.

V4 H: "Does your baby respond to your facial expressions?"

V4 T: Engage baby's gaze and attempt to elicit a smile by smiling and talking to baby. Then scowl at baby. Pass if any change in baby's facial expression.

V5 T: Horizontal (H): Engage child's gaze with yours at a distance of 18 inches. Move slowly back and forth. Pass if child turns head 60° to the left and right from midline. Vertical (V): Move slowly up and down. Pass if child elevates eyes 30° from horizontal. Must pass both H and V to pass item.

V6 T: Flick your fingers rapidly toward child's face, ending with fingertips 1 to 2 inches from face. Do not touch face or eyelashes. Pass if child blinks.

V7 H: Does child play pat-a-cake, peek-a-boo, etc., in response to parents?

V8 T: See note for AR8 (always try AR8 first; if AR8 is passed, then automatically give credit for V8).

V9 H: Does child spontaneously initiate gesture games?

V10 H: "Does your child ever point with index finger to something wanted? For example, if child is sitting at the dinner table and wants something that is out of reach, how does child let you know what is wanted?" Pass *only* index finger pointing, *not* reaching with whole hand.

EARLY LANGUAGE MILESTONE SCALE (ELM) SCALE: UPDATE—JUNE 1987

The Early Language Milestone Scale (ELM Scale) was introduced into clinical practice in 1983. Since that time, the ELM Scale has been used successfully in a variety of settings, including well-child clinics, neonatal intensive care follow-up programs, public school screening programs, and doctors' offices.

The purpose of this communication is to acquaint you with one significant addition and several minor revisions that have recently been incorporated into the Auditory Expressive division of the ELM Scale.

The biggest change has been the addition of a new item cluster pertaining to intelligibility of speech. The Auditory Expressive division of the ELM Scale now consists of two parts: Content (cooing, babbling, use of words, phrases, etc.) and Intelligibility. This Intelligibility Cluster has been added in response to requests from users of the ELM Scale because many children seen for evaluation of "delayed speech" have unclear (unintelligible) speech.

Administration of Intelligibility Cluster

The Intelligibility Cluster contains three bars:

AE15: "About half"
AE19: "Three quarters"
AE20: "All or almost all"

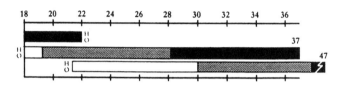

All three items may be scored by asking the parent the following forced-choice question:

"How clear is your child's speech? That is, how much of your child's speech can a stranger understand: Less than half, about half, three quarters, or all or almost all?"

Parents or other adults in close contact with a child often become attuned to the child's speech pattern, including any distortions of speech-sound production. Parents, therefore, are *not* the best ones to judge the intelligibility of their own child's speech. This is why the parent is asked to guess how clear the child sounds to *others*: "How much of your child's speech can a *stranger* understand . . . ?" The wording *must* be followed when eliciting the parent's response.

Scoring

If parents report that "less than half" of the child's speech can be understood by strangers, child fails all three items in Intelligibility Cluster.

If "about half" of child's speech can be understood by strangers, child passes AE15 ("about half") but fails AE 19 ("three quarters") and AE20 ("all or almost all").

If "three quarters" of child's speech can be understood by strangers, child passes both AE15 ("about half") and AE19 ("three quarters") but fails AE20 ("all or almost all").

If "all or almost all" of child's speech can be understood by strangers, child passes all three items in Intelligibility Cluster.

If the child fails to attain intelligibility at a level equal to that already attained by 90% or more of children of the same age, then the child fails the Intelligibility Cluster and the ELM Scale as a whole.

When to Administer the Intelligibility Cluster

The Intelligibility Cluster should be administered to all children 18 months of age or older. It should be administered *in addition* to the three or more items required to obtain a basal level in the Content portion of the Auditory Expressive division. A child greater than 18 months must pass both the Intelligibility Cluster *and* the Content portion of the Auditory Expressive division to pass the Auditory Expressive division as a whole.

Special Cases

1. Some children over the age of 18 months may not be scorable in the Intelligibility Cluster because they are not producing any words, intelligible or otherwise. Such children all fail the ELM Scale because of their delay in the appearance of speech, since the 90% value for the emergence of single words is approximately 17.5 months.
2. The primary age range of the ELM Scale is from birth to 36 months. Note that the 90% value for item AE19 is 37 months, and for item AE20 is 47 months. Since the ELM Scale is often used with children over 36 months whose speech or language are delayed, these age values are displayed for convenience at the right edge of the bar for these two items.

Other Revisions to ELM Scale

Two items have been eliminated: old item AE15 (correct use of "me" and "you") and old item AE19 (correct use of the pronoun "I"). This should produce minimal effect on scoring: Old item AE15 (correct use of "me" and "you") was represented by a place holder on the first edition of the ELM Scale and was not used in scoring the Scale. The 90% value for old item AE19 (correct use of the pronoun "I") extended well above 36 months of age. Therefore, the child's performance on this item was unlikely to determine whether the child passed or failed the ELM Scale as a whole. Note that the item *numbers* AE15 and AE19 have been reassigned to two of the three bars in the Intelligibility Cluster. All of the other Auditory Expressive items stay in the same sequence as on the first edition of the ELM Scale, with the same number designations as before.

Index